CONTENTS

rilling is a great way to cook delicious and healthy meals as well as enjoy the outdoors. For many eople, grilling food is also very beneficial as it can help lower calorie intake thus may help with weight ss. While grilling does not necessarily remove all fats from meat, it allows extra fat to melt and drip off nd not get reabsorbed. Moreover, grilling also helps seal in vitamins and minerals, unlike other ooking methods. However, many people opt not to use this cooking method because of the misnomer at the food that they are going to cook will be limited to charred meats. Fortunately, grilling will never estrict you to cooking meat alone. With the right griller, you will also be able to bake, broil, and even ake casseroles. This is where the Pit Boss Wood Pellet Grill comes in.

Why Pit Boss Wood Pellet Grill?

he Pit Boss Wood Pellet Grill is the latest buzz in the BBQ world and it uses wood pellets to grill your od thus adding extra kick, flavor, and dimension to your food. Unlike conventional charcoal grills, this articular grill requires you to use compressed pellets and feed them into the grill's fire pot to heat the rill to the desired temperature. Having said this, wood pellet grills allow you more control over the emperature settings of your grill. This prevents you from charring or overcooking your good. Plus, you on't need to babysit your grill at all times compared to your usual charcoal grill. Since you don't need watch over the grill at all times, you now have more time for entertaining. Isn't this what grilling is all bout?

enefits Of Pit Boss Wood Pellet Grill

you are contemplating on replacing your old charcoal grill, then now is the time to do it. The Pit Boss Vood Pellet Grill comes with a lot of benefits that you will never enjoy with your conventional charcoal rill.

- **Effortless ignition:** To light your wood pellet grill, you don't need accelerants like lighter fluid to start a fire. Simply prime the fire pot and ignite the grill with a mere touch of a button. The intuitive controller of the grill will take care of everything for you.
- **Even heat:** Wood pellet grills provide generally even heat throughout every nook and cranny of the grill this means that you can place your food anywhere in the grill and everything will cook at the same time. It comes with a PID (Proportional, Integral, Derivative) Controller that adds complexity to the temperature control method. With this controller, you will not only have a better control temperature range, but you also have the capacity to monitor the smoke produced, track your pellet consumption, and monitor your meat without the need to open the grill.
- **Wireless connectivity:** The Pit Boss Wood Pellet Grill is a smart kitchen device that will make your life so much easier! It comes with a phone app that you can control via Wi-Fi or

Bluetooth so that you can control the grill from your smartphone even if you are out on a grocery run.

- **Great smoke flavor:** Wood BBQ pellets come in a myriad of flavors from hickory, pecan, maple,
- cherry, and many others. You also have the freedom to mix different flavors to make your food more interesting. These wood pellets are not only great in adding another layer of flavor to your meats but they will definitely make your baked goods more interesting.
- **Comes with pre-programmed cooking cycles:** To make your grilling easier, the Pit Boss Wood Pellet Grill comes with pre-programmed smoking cycles. This removes the guesswork when cooking different kinds of foods.
- **Cooks all kinds of foods:** Wood pellet grills are capable of cooking just about all kinds of foods. You can grill, BBQ, smoke, bake, broil, and even sear. It is one of the few kitchen devices that you can truly call an all-in-one cooking machine.

Why The Pit Boss Wood Pellet Grill Is Your Better Option

First introduced in the market in 1999, the Pit Boss Wood Pellet Grill has been around for more than two decades to make grilling easier and more convenient to many people. While it is still a fairly new brand compared to its older counterparts, this brand of wood pellet grill is very dependable. Although reviews online would put the Pit Boss Wood Pellet Grill second to its biggest competitor, Traeger Grill, in terms of size and portability, it is my firm belief that there are still so many benefits that make the Pit Boss Wood Pellet Grill worthy of your time and bucks.

- **More affordable:** If you are looking for a line of wood pellet grills that are affordable, the Pit Boss Wood Pellet Grill comes with affordable options. You don't need to shell out a lot of money to buy this kitchen appliance. Their wood pellet grills have a price range of $390 to $2490 depending on the capacity of the grill. This is an extremely cheaper option compared to other wood pellet grills that start at $500 and above.
- **Simpler interface and parts:** The manufacturer of the Pit Boss Wood Pellet Grill banks on simplicity as its main selling point. It comes with an intuitive user interface that makes it so easy to control. Moreover, it also comes with fewer parts that make it very easy to assemble.
- **Uses relevant technologies:** Modern Pit Boss Wood Pellet Grills come with relevant technology. These include remote settings using Bluetooth and Wi-Fi specifically on its Platinum line of grills.
- **Built-in working station:** The Pit Boss Pellet Grill comes with a built-in working station including built-in tool hooks and a solid side shelf. This makes it a perfect kitchen appliance that you can put in any part of your outdoor space. When it comes to movability, it may not be as portable as other brands of wood pellet grills but it comes with locking caster wheels that will allow you to push the grill anywhere and keep it in place. Its reinforced leg design makes it a sturdy wood grill for heavy-duty cooking.

Wood Pellet Guide For Grilling

Understanding your many options for wood pellets for grilling is crucial for you to maximize your cooking experience with our Pit Boss Wood Pellet Grill. In fact, choosing the right wood pellet is the heart and soul of cooking with your wood pellet grill. Wood pellets are basically the main fuel source of the grill. They are made from 100% natural hardwood that is dried, grounds, and manipulated to equally sized pellets using extreme heat and pressure. There are two types of wood pellets that are available in the market: heating pellets and food-grade pellets. Heating pellets are made from wood that is not meant for smoking your meats and they are made together with glue and other additives that are not good for your food. Examples of heating pellets include those made from spruce and pine.

Thus, when buying wood pellets for your Pit Boss Wood Pellet Grill, make sure to look for the food-grade pellets as they do not contain binders and additives. Moreover, they also impart interesting flavor to your food making them more interesting and delicious. Food-grade pellets include mesquite, hickory, cherry, pecan, apple, oak, and alder. And so, the proverbial question *which food-grade pellet goes well with what food?"*

- **Competition blend:** Comes with a smoky and sweet aromatic tang. It is made from a blend of hickory, maple, and cherry thus it comes with a soft fruity undertone. This is perfect for beef, pork, chicken, fish, veggies, fruits, and desserts.
- **Hickory:** Comes with a rich bacon-like flavor and is great for roasts and smoking meats.
- **Mesquite:** This wood pellet comes with a strong aroma with a hint of tangy and spicy flavor. This is a great wood pellet for those who enjoy Tex-Mex cuisines.
- **Apple:** This comes with a mildly sweet and smoky flavor and is great for pork and baking desserts.
- **Classic:** Comes with a bold blend of mesquite, hickory, and pecan that imparts a full-bodied flavor that can bring out the best in any chicken, pork, veggies, and seafood.
- **Fruit:** This blend of wood pellets imparts an all-natural fruity undertone thus making it great for pork and baking. Surprisingly, it also works well with poultry and seafood.
- **Charcoal blend:** Comes with a bold aroma of oak and a smoky hint of charcoal. This is a great blend for beef, pork, game, and poultry.

When it comes to choosing the right wood pellet for your grill, make sure that you opt for quality brand pellets. Getting a cheaply made brand will not only ruin your food but can also damage the inner workings of your pellet grill. Fortunately, the Pit Boss Wood Pellet Grill has its own brand of wood pellets to choose from.

Grilling Tips For Beginners

Grilling and smoking your food using the Pit Boss Wood Pellet Grill is no rocket science. However, if it is your first time using a wood pellet grill, below are great tips that you can help as a beginner.

- **Know your meat:** Different kinds of meats require different grilling settings. When choosing meat for grilling, you need to know the composition (fat to muscle ratio, cartilage, bones) of your meat, color, and texture. Different cuts of meats need to be treated in different ways. For instance, lean cuts such as chicken breasts dry out easily compared with red meat.
- **Always brine your meat:** To impart flavor and moisture to your meat, you can brine your meat in advance prior to grilling or smoking.
- **Do not flip your meat all the time:** The Pit Boss Wood Pellet Grill is unlike your open charcoal grill. Flipping the meat means that you need to open the grill and this will reduce the internal temperature inside the cooking chamber. Only flip the meat once. In fact, you don't even need to do it since all sides can cook evenly.
- **Get the right accessories:** The Pit Boss Wood Pellet Grill comes with many types of accessories that you can use to maximize your grilling and smoking experience. You can get skillet pans, side shelf, iron griddle, iron roaster, meat hooks.

Starting Up Your Grill

Starting up the Pit Boss Wood Pellet Grill is as simple as plugging it in and turning your temperature dial. While it sounds as easy as it seems, there are some things that you need to take note of.

1. **Place fuel in the hopper:** The fuel of your grill is the wood pellet. Make sure that you have at least 2 pounds of pellets for every hour of smoking. If you are going to grill, you need 4 pounds for every hour of fast grilling.
2. **Set the grill to smoke and open the lid:** Open the hood of the grill and set it to smoke. This is an important step as it gives the igniter the chance to light before feeding more wood pellets. Oxygen is needed for the igniter to light. If the lid is closed, it will not line up and the pellets will merely line up in the pot and may eventually spill over the cooking chamber. This usually takes about three minutes to light up.
3. **Watch out for thick smoke:** When you notice that there is thick smoke billowing out of the grill, this means that your pot has caught and that your pellets are burning. Fortunately, the Pit Boss Wood Pellet Grill can fix this problem on its own. Allow the smoke to billow out from the grill for 4 minutes and it will eventually dissipate.
4. **Crank up and start grilling:** Once the pot catches, the convection fan will start blowing on the flame inside the grill. You can then crank up the temperature so that you can start grilling. You can close the lid so that the heat will climb to the desired temperature.

BEEF RECIPES

Grilled Hanger Steak Pinwheels

Servings: 4
Cooking Time: 30 Minutes
Ingredients:

- 2 Tablespoons Chophouse Steak Seasoning
- Zest From 2 Lemons
- ¾ Cup Finely Parsley, Chopped
- 1 Pkg Provolone Cheese, Sliced
- 6 Oz Washed Spinach
- 1 Whole 1 ½ Pound Trimmed Hanger, Skirt, Or Steak, Flank

Directions:

1. Cut the steak into two even size pieces. Lay the steak out on a flat work surface and cover with plastic wrap. Using a meat mallet, gently pound the steak until it's at least 4 inches wide and no more than 1/3 inch thick.
2. Season both sides of each steak with Chophouse Seasoning. Lay the provolone cheese first followed by spinach. Beginning at the thinnest end of the steak, roll the steak up around the filling. Repeat with the second steak.
3. Tie a length of butcher's twin around the middle, then one piece around the ends. Cut the rolls in half, then slice the wheels again at the twine. Repeat this process with the second steak.
4. Fire up your Pit Boss and set the temperature to 400°F. If you're using a gas or charcoal grill, set it up for high heat.
5. Cook the pinwheels cut-side down, flipping once, or until browned on both sides and cooked to your liking, about 10-15 minutes each side for medium rare (135°F). Let the pinwheels rest for 5 minutes before serving.

Spicy Chopped Brisket Sandwich With Sauce And Jalapeno

Servings: 4
Cooking Time: 10 Minutes
Ingredients:

- 3 Cups Cooked And Chopped Brisket
- Dill Pickle, Slice
- Pickled Jalapeno, Sliced
- 4 Sandwich Buns
- 1 Cup Spicy Barbecue Sauce
- White Onion, Sliced

Directions:

1. Fire up your Pit Boss and set the temperature to 350°F. If you're using gas or charcoal, prep your grill to cook with medium indirect heat.
2. Add the chopped brisket and spicy barbecue sauce to the aluminum pan and mix well. The brisket should be fully coated with sauce. If 1 cup is not enough, feel free to more sauce ¼ cup at a time.
3. Cover the aluminum pan tightly with foil and place it in the center of the grill. Close the lid and cook the brisket for about 10 minutes or until it's heated all the way through.
4. Remove the brisket from the grill and pile the meat on top of the sandwich buns. Top the brisket sandwich with pickle slices, jalapeno slices, and sliced onions. Serve immediately.

Tomahawk Steak With Apple Butter

Servings: 2 – 4
Cooking Time: 215 Minutes

Ingredients:

- Apple Corer Or Metal Spoon
- 3 Lbs Gala Apples
- 1 Lemon
- Pit Boss Chop House Steak Rub
- 1 Tbsp Pit Boss Tennessee Apple Butter Rub
- Sugar
- 4 Cups Water

Directions:

1. Fire up your Pit Boss and preheat to 400°F. If using a gas or charcoal grill, set heat to medium-high heat.
2. Core and halve the apples. Place apples skin-side down on a sheet tray and season with Tennessee Apple Butter and set aside.
3. In a cast iron pot, combine the apple cores with the juice and zest from one lemon. Cover the mixture with water, transfer to the grill and bring to a boil. Reduce heat to 225° F. Place the apples directly on the grill grate (skin-side down) and cook for 1 hour.
4. After 1 hour, remove cast iron pot from the grill. Strain liquid, discard cores, return liquid to pot, and whisk in sugar. Cover with lid and return to grill. Allow to simmer for another hour.
5. Add smoked apples to the pot and continue to simmer for 20 minutes. Remove pot from grill and purée apple mixture in a blender. Pour apple purée back into pot and return to grill. Increase heat to 375° F and simmer for 20 minutes. Remove from grill and allow to cool slightly.
6. Reduce heat on grill to 225° F. Season the tomahawk steak with Pit Boss Chop House Steak Rub on both sides. Place the steak on the grill grates, insert a temperature probe, and grill, undisturbed, for 45 minutes, or until the steak reaches an internal temperature of 120°F
7. Remove steak from grill and set aside. Open the Sear Slide on your Pit Boss and increase temperature to 400°F. Return tomahawk to grill and sear over open flames, about 2-3 minutes per side.
8. Pull the steak off the grill and allow it to rest for 10 minutes. Ladle reserved apple butter over steak and serve.

Cowboy Nachos

Servings: 8
Cooking Time: 20 Minutes

Ingredients:

- Cilantro
- Olive Oil
- Pepper
- 1 Red Bell Peppers, Sliced
- 2 Rib-Eye Steaks
- Salsa
- Salt
- 1 Cup Shredded Cheddar Cheese
- Sour Cream
- 1 Yellow Bell Pepper, Sliced
- 1 Zucchini, Sliced

Directions:

1. Preheat your grill to 400°F.
2. Coat both sides of the steak with olive oil and season with sea salt and pepper. Place the steak on the grates and grill for about 4 to 5 minutes per side.
3. Remove the steak off the grill and let rest for about 10 minutes before cutting into bite-sized strips.
4. Brush with barbecue sauce if desired.
5. Empty a large bag of nacho chips evenly into a cast iron pan. Start loading up with toppings - steak, cheddar cheese, sautéed vegetables.

6. These are just suggested toppings, so feel free to add anything you like!

7. Place your loaded nachos on the grill and let the hot smoke melt your toppings into one hearty creation.

8. Cook for about 10 minutes, or until the cheese has fully melted.

9. Remove and serve with sour cream and salsa.

Burnt Ends

Servings: 10-12
Cooking Time: 1440 Minutes
Ingredients:
- 1 Cup Apple Cider Vinegar
- 1 Jar Barbecue Sauce
- 1/2 (Any Brand) Beer, Can
- Pit Boss Beef And Brisket Rub
- 10 - 12 Pound Whole Beef Brisket
- 2 Tablespoons Worcestershire Sauc

Directions:
1. Remove the brisket from the refrigerator. Trimming a cold brisket is easier than trimming a room temperature brisket. Flip the brisket over so that the pointed end of the meat is facing under. Cut away any silver skin or excess fat from the flat muscle and discard. Next, there will be a large, crescent shaped fat section on the flat of the meat. Trim that fat until it is smooth against the meat so that it looks like a seamless transition between the point and flat. Flip the brisket over and trim the fat cap to ¼ inch thick.

2. Generously season the trimmed brisket on all sides with the Pit Boss Beef and Brisket Seasoning.

3. In a bowl, mix together the beer (for a gluten free brisket, be sure to use GF beer), apple cider vinegar and Worcestershire sauce to make mop sauce.

4. Preheat your Pit Boss Smoker to 225°F. Place the brisket in the smoker, insert a temperature probe, and smoke until the internal temperature reads 165°F, about 8 hours. Baste the brisket with the mop sauce every 2 hours to keep it moist. Once the brisket reaches 165°F, remove from the smoker, wrap in butcher paper, folding the edges over to form a leak proof seal, and return to the smoker seam-side down for another 5-8 hours, or until the brisket reaches 202°F.

5. Remove from the smoker, place in an insulated cooler, and allow to rest for 3 hours. Once the brisket has finished resting, heat your Pit Boss smoker to 275°F. Unwrap the brisket and cut the flat from the point. Re wrap the flat and save for another recipe. Cut the point into chunks, coat in barbecue sauce, and sprinkle with Beef and Brisket seasoning.

6. Smoke the burnt ends for 1 hour, or until deeply burnished and glazed. Serve and enjoy!

Barbecue Beef Brisket

Servings: 12
Cooking Time: 480 Minutes
Ingredients:
- 1 Beef Soup, Campbells Can
- 1 - 12 To 14 Lb Packer Beef, Brisket

Directions:
1. The night before you plan on cooking the brisket, trim the surface fat off the brisket with your sharp boning knife. Trim to leave about 1/8 to ¼ in fat.

2. Place the brisket in an unscented trash bag or on a sheet pan fat side up and season the meat side liberally with your favorite Rub. Let rest on the counter for 30 minutes until the rub is all soaked up. Flip the brisket over and season the fat side liberally. Cover or wrap up the brisket and put in the fridge overnight.

3. Prep your Grill by cleaning the grates, grease tray and firepot is clean. Start the grill and set to 250°F.

4. When grill has settled to 250°F place brisket in center of grill fat side down and cook for 4 hours.

5. After 4 hours, insert the meat probe into the fat seam between the point and flat so the end of the meat probe is in the center of the fat seam and continue to cook for about 2 more hours.

6. Prep aluminum foil to wrap the brisket in by tearing off 4 sheets of foil at least twice as large as the brisket. Plus one more piece about the same size as the brisket.

7. When the meat thermometer reads 150°F to 160°F wrap the brisket in foil by placing the brisket fat side down on 2 sheets of foil. The cover with the other 2 sheets of foil and tightly roll/fold 3 sides up to seal – leaving one side open. Leave the meat probe in place in the brisket and lay the probe wire between the bottom and top foil sheets. Roll/fold the meat probe wire between the foil sheets as you are closing the foil. Dump the can of Campbell's Beef Consume into the foil through the open end and roll/fold that end closed.

8. Place the small foil sheet on the grill grate and place the foil-wrapped brisket on the small foil sheet on the grate. The small foil sheet will prevent the foil from sticking to the grate to prevent the foil from ripping and losing the foil juice that you can use later.

9. Continue to cook until the meat thermometer reads 200°F. Then unwrap one or two sides of the foil being careful not to lose any of the liquid in the foil. Insert a dinner fork into the flat portion of the brisket – if it goes in and out like a hot knife through butter it is done, if it has very much resistance, seal the sides of the foil and place back in grill and cook until

the meat thermometer reads 205°F and test for tenderness again.

10. When the brisket is done, remove from grill, wrap in a clean towel and place in a small clean cooler to rest for at least 2 hours.

11. When ready to slice, remove brisket from foil. Separate the point end from the flat end by running your slicing knife down the fat seam. Slice the brisket across the grain into slices just thick enough to hold together.

12. Cube the point section into ½ in sq cubes by slicing ½ in slices across the grain first and then ½ in slices with the grain.

13. Place all slices and cubes into a pan and pour some of the liquid from the foil over the brisket.

14. Serve with your favorite BBQ Sauce on the side.

Smoked Meatball Sandwiches

Servings: 4
Cooking Time: 25 Minutes
Ingredients:

- 3/4 Cup Breadcrumbs
- 2 Cloves Garlic, Minced
- 1 & 1/2 Lb. Ground Chuck
- 1 Jar Of Your Favorite Marinara Sauce
- 1 Large Eggs
- ¼ Cup Onion
- ¼ Cup Parsley, Minced Fresh
- ½ Tsp Pepper
- 1 Tbsp Pit Boss Chop House Steak Seasoning
- Provolone Cheese, Sliced
- ½ Tsp Salt
- Shredded Mozzarella Cheese
- 4 Sub Rolls Or Baguettes (6"), Sliced
- 2 Tbsp Worcestershire

Directions:

1. In a larger mixing bowl, combine the ground chuck, onions, garlic, Chop House Steak seasoning, salt, pepper, fresh parsley, Worcestershire, and egg. Add the breadcrumb mixture and parmesan cheese to the bowl and fold it into meat until well combined.

2. Fire up your Pit Boss Grill to "smoke" with the lid open until a fire is established in the burn pot, 3-7 minutes. Preheat to 400°F. If you're using a gas or charcoal grill, set it up for medium high heat and add your cast iron pan to the grill to warm up.

3. Roll the meat mixture into balls about 1 ½ inches wide, roughly the size of golf balls. Place meatballs into the cast iron skillet. Cook for 15 minutes or until meatballs are fully cooked and beginning to brown.

4. Pour full jar of marinara into the cast iron pan and gently stir to coat meatballs. Let simmer for 10-15 minutes.

5. Tear off four sheets of aluminum foil and place a sliced bun in the center of each. Divide the meatballs with sauce among the rolls. Top each roll with provolone cheese slices and mozzarella, and wrap entire sandwich tightly in foil. Return to the grill and cook an additional 10 minutes or until cheese is melty and bread has toasted. Serve immediately and enjoy!

Smoked Beef Caldereta Stew

Servings: 12
Cooking Time:240 Mins
Ingredients:

- 1/2 cup cheddar cheese, grated
- 2 lbs, cut into 1 1/2" cubes chuck roast
- 4 garlic cloves, chopped
- 1 tsp kosher salt
- 2 tbsp olive oil
- 2 large yukon gold potatoes
- 5 chopped serrano peppers

- 2 tbsp tomato paste
- 2 cups tomato sauce
- 2 cups water

Directions:

1. Place beef in a cast iron skillet, then transfer to smoking cabinet. Make sure that the sear slide and side dampers are open, then increase temperature to 375°F, to ensure the cabinet maintains temperature between 225°F and 250°F (If you're cooking on a different Pit Boss Pellet Grill, set the temperature to 225°F).

2. Smoke beef for 1½ hours, then turn cubed beef, and smoke an additional 1½ hours.

3. Place cast iron Dutch oven on the grill, over flame. Add olive oil, potatoes, and carrots. Cook for 3 to 5 minutes, stirring occasionally. Then add leeks and garlic and cook for 2 minutes, until fragrant.

4. Remove skillet from smoking cabinet and add beef pieces to potato mixture.

5. Add tomato sauce, tomato paste, water, and serrano peppers. Bring to a boil, then cover with lid. Set temperature to 275°F, and allow stew to simmer for 1 hour, until beef and potatoes are tender.

6. Add liver and cheese, and gently stir to combine, until the sauce thickens and cheese has melted.

7. Add bell peppers and olives. Stir, cover and cook an additional 2 minutes. Season with salt, and serve hot.

Tri Tip Burnt Ends

Servings: 3
Cooking Time:420mins
Ingredients:

- 1/2 cup bbq sauce
- to taste, beef & brisket rub
- 1 1/2 tbsp brown sugar
- 1 1/2 tbsp butter, cubed
- 1/2 cup dr. pepper soda
- 1/2 tbsp honey

- 2 tbsp mustard
- 2 lbs tri tip steak
- 1/2 tbsp worcestershire sauce

Directions:

1. Fire up your Pit Boss Platinum Series KC Combo on SMOKE mode and let it run with lid open for 10 minutes then set it to 225° F. If using a gas or charcoal grill, set it up for low, indirect heat.
2. Rub the mustard all over the tri tip, then season with Beef & Brisket rub.
3. Place the tri tip directly on the grill grates and smoke until the internal temperature reaches 165° F (about 2 1/2 hours).
4. Remove the tri tip from the grill and wrap it in Pit Boss butcher paper. Return the tri tip to the grill and continue to smoke until the internal temperature reaches 200° F (an additional 2 ½ to 3 hours).
5. Remove the tri tip from the grill, and rest for 30 minutes, or rest and refrigerate overnight.
6. Increase the grill temperature to 275° F.
7. Cube into ½ inch to ¾ inch pieces, then place cubed tri tip in a large cast iron skillet.
8. Stir together BBQ sauce, Dr. Pepper, honey, and worcestershire sauce in a jar or mixing bowl, then pour over the cubed tri tip. Dot with butter, then sprinkle brown sugar over the top.
9. Place skillet on the grill grate, over indirect heat. Cook for 1 ½ to 2 hours, rotating pieces halfway through cooking. Sauce will have reduced, coated and slightly char the tri tip. Remove from the grill and serve warm.

Reverse Seared Bacon Wrapped Steaks

Servings: 2
Cooking Time: 60 Minutes
Ingredients:

- 1 Bunch Asparagus
- 4 Bacon, Strip
- Bbq Sauce
- 2 Tbsp Olive Oil
- 1 Bag Potato, Baby
- 2 - 1" Thick Steak, Bone-In Ribeye

Directions:

1. Start your Grill on "smoke" with the lid open until a fire is established in the burn pot (3-7 minutes). Preheat to 250°F.
2. Wrap two pieces of bacon around each steak. Place on the grates of your preheated Grill. You'll want to cook the steaks until the internal temperature reaches 130°F (for medium-rare). Follow these internal temperatures if you'd like to cook your steak more/less done:
3. Rare: 125°F
4. Medium Rare: 130°F
5. Medium: 140°F
6. Well Done: 160°F
7. If you're cooking your steaks medium rare it will take around 45 minutes. Put your baby potatoes in a cast iron pan, drizzle with oil and place on grill with the steaks. When your steaks reach the desired internal temperature, remove steaks from the grill and let them rest for 15 minutes. In the meantime, open up your Flame Broiler Plate and crank up the grill to HIGH, keeping your potatoes on the grill. Add the asparagus to the top of the potatoes and cook. When the grill is preheated to HIGH, sear each side of the steak for about 1 minute each. Serve immediately with or without BBQ Sauce.

Pigs In A Blanket

Servings: 10
Cooking Time: 15 Minutes
Ingredients:

- 1 Crescent Dough, Can
- 1 Egg

- 1 Tsp Garlic, Minced
- 20 Hot Dog, Mini
- 1/4 Cup Mustard, Dijon
- 1 Tbsp Onion, Diced
- 2 Tbsp Poppy Seeds
- 1 Tsp Salt, Coarse

Directions:

1. Turn on your and preheat to 350°F. Combine the poppy seeds, dried minced onion, minced garlic, and salt in a bowl.
2. Unroll the crescent roll dough, pull apart the triangles and slice each segment into three little triangle pieces. Try to get 3 strips for each roll for the mini hot dogs.
3. After the strips are cut, spread some Dijon mustard on each piece of dough. Roll the dough around mini hot dogs. Lay the pigs in a blanket on a greased cookie sheet. Brush with egg wash and sprinkle with the prepared seasoning.
4. Bake for 15 minutes, serve hot and enjoy!

Reverse Seared T-bone Steak

Servings: 1 - 2
Cooking Time: 64 Minutes
Ingredients:

- Pit Boss Java Chop House Rub
- 1 Steak, T-Bone

Directions:

1. Preheat your Pit Boss Grill to 250°F then close the lid 10-15 minutes.
2. As the is preheating to the perfect temperature, spice the T-bone with your favorite steak rub.
3. Lay the steak on the grill for roughly 60 minutes or until the steaks reach an internal temperature of 105 to 110°F. Remove the steaks and set aside.
4. Crank up the heat to 450°F and open the flame broiler.
5. Place the steak over the flame broiler and sear for about 2 minutes a side, 4 minutes in total. You know when your steak is done

once the internal temperature reaches 130 to 135°F (for medium-rare). Follow the below internal temperature for your cooking preference:

6. Rare: 125°F
7. Medium Rare: 130°F
8. Medium: 140°F
9. Well Done: 160°F
10. Once reached for personal preference, take the steaks off the grill and eat! Enjoy!

Texas Style Smoked Brisket

Servings:10-12
Cooking Time:480 Mins
Ingredients:

- 1 cup apple cider vinegar
- 1/2 (any brand) beer, can
- pit boss beef and brisket rub
- 10-12 pound whole beef brisket
- 2 tablespoons worcestershire sauce

Directions:

1. Remove the brisket from the refrigerator. Trimming a cold brisket is easier than trimming a room temperature brisket.
2. Flip the brisket over so that the pointed end of the meat is facing under. Cut away any silver skin or excess fat from the flat muscle and discard.
3. Next, there will be a large, crescent shaped fat section on the flat of the meat. Trim that fat until it is smooth against the meat so that it looks like a seamless transition between the point and flat.
4. Flip the brisket over and trim the fat cap to ¼ inch thick.
5. Generously season the trimmed brisket on all sides with the Pit Boss Beef and Brisket Seasoning.
6. In a bowl, mix together the beer, apple cider vinegar and Worcestershire sauce to make mop sauce.
7. Preheat your Pit Boss Smoker to 225°F.

8. Place the brisket in the smoker, insert a temperature probe, and smoke until the internal temperature reads 165°F, about 8 hours.
9. Baste the brisket with the mop sauce every 2 hours to keep it moist.
10. Once the brisket reaches 165F, remove from the smoker, wrap in butcher paper, folding the edges over to form a leakproof seal, and return to the smoker seam-side down for another 5-8 hours, or until the brisket is tender enough to slide in a probe with little to no effort (around 203°F).
11. Remove the brisket from the smoker and allow to rest for 1 hour before slicing.

Philly Cheese Steaks

Servings: 6
Cooking Time: 45 Minutes
Ingredients:
- 2 Green Bell Pepper, Sliced
- 6 Hot Dog Bun(S)
- 2 Cups Mozzarella Cheese, Shredded
- 1 Quart Mushroom
- 1 Onion, Sliced
- Pepper
- Salt
- 2 Thick Steak, Flank

Directions:
1. Start your Grill on SMOKE with the lid open until a fire is established in the burn pot (10 minutes).
2. Preheat to 250°F.
3. Season both sides of your steaks with salt and pepper to your liking. We're going to reverse sear these steaks, so place on the grates of your preheated Grill. You'll want to cook the steaks until the internal temperature reaches 130°F (for medium-rare). Follow these internal temperatures if you'd like to cook your steak more/less done:
4. Rare: 125°F

5. Medium Rare: 130°F
6. Medium: 140°F
7. Well Done: 160°F
8. If you're cooking your steaks medium rare it will take around 45 minutes depending on how thick the steaks are.
9. While the steaks are cooking, slice up the onion, mushrooms, and peppers thinly and sauté until soft.
10. When the steaks have reached your desired internal temperature, remove steaks from the grill and let them rest for 15 minutes. In the meantime, open up your flame broiler and crank up the grill to HIGH. Sear each side of the steak for about 1 minutes each.
11. Rest steaks again for 10 minutes.
12. Slice steak thinly, combine with the sautéed vegetables and fill a hot dog bun generously with the mixture.

Smoked Beef Back Ribs

Servings:2 – 4
Cooking Time:260mins
Ingredients:
- 2 racks beef back ribs
- ½ tbsp black pepper
- ⅓ cup pit boss chop house steak seasoning

Directions:
1. Fire up your Pit Boss and preheat pellet grill to 250°F. If using a gas or charcoal grill, set it up for low heat.
2. Place the ribs on a sheet tray, then remove the membrane from the back of the ribs: Take a butter knife and wedge it just underneath the membrane to loosen it. Using your hands, or a paper towel to grip, pull the membrane up and off the bone. Rub each rack generously with Pit Boss Chop House Steak seasoning and black pepper.
3. Place the ribs on the grill and smoke for 2 hours. Increase the temperature to 300°F

and cook an additional 45 to 60 minutes, or until the ribs reach an internal temperature of 205° F. Be sure and flip the ribs halfway to achieve good bark.

4. Remove ribs from the grill and wrap in butcher paper. Allow ribs to rest for 20 minutes, then slice and serve hot.

Bison Meatballs With Cider Mustard Sauce

Servings: 8 - 10
Cooking Time: 30 Minutes
Ingredients:

- 1 Cored, Peeled, And Chopped Apple
- 2 Tablespoons Beef & Brisket Rub
- 2 Cups Beef Broth
- 2 Pounds Ground Bison
- ¼ Cup Breadcrumbs
- 3 Tablespoons Cornstarch
- 2 Tablespoons Dijon Mustard
- 2 Beaten Eggs
- 1 Finely Garlic Clove, Minced
- 2 Cups Hard Cider
- 3 Tablespoons Pure Maple Syrup
- 2 Tablespoons Olive Oil
- ½ Cup Pureed Onion
- ¼ Pound Pancetta
- 3 Tablespoons Water
- 1 Thinly Sliced Yellow Onion

Directions:

1. First, make the mustard sauce. In a large saucepan, add the olive oil over medium heat, then add the onion and apple. Cook the apple and onion until soft and caramelized, about 10-12 minutes. Once the onion and apple are soft, add in the hard cider, beef broth, maple syrup and Dijon mustard to the pan. Whisk everything together and bring the sauce to a boil.

2. Once the sauce comes to a boil, reduce it to a simmer and cook, stirring and scraping the bottom of the pot occasionally until the sauce reduces by half, about 30 minutes. Remove the sauce from the heat and allow it to cool.

3. Pour the sauce into a blender, place the lid on top, and blend the sauce until completely smooth. Return the sauce into the saucepan and bring it back to a boil. In a small bowl, mix together the cornstarch and water, then pour into the sauce. Cook the sauce until thickened, whisking the entire time, about 2 minutes. Set the sauce aside.

4. Make the meatballs. In a food processor, blend the pancetta until it becomes a smooth paste. Scrape the pancetta into large mixing bowl, and mix it with the ground bison, pureed onion, eggs, breadcrumbs, garlic, and Beef and Brisket Rub. Gently mix the meat together and, using a cookie scoop, scoop into meatballs. Place the meatballs on a baking sheet. Repeat with the remaining meat mixture.

5. Fire up your Pit Boss and set the temperature to 350°F. If you're using a gas or charcoal grill, set it up for medium heat. Place a large cast iron skillet on the grill and add the olive oil to it. Place the meatballs in an even layer in the skillet and grill, turning the meatballs occasionally until they are browned on all sides. Insert a temperature probe into one of the meatballs and continue grilling them until the internal temperature reaches 160°F.

6. Remove the meatballs from the grill, toss them with the mustard sauce, and serve immediately.

Texas Twinkies

Servings:7-14
Cooking Time:40mins
Ingredients:

- 14, slices bacon

23

- ½ cup bbq sauce
- 1 lb. brisket
- 8 oz. cream cheese
- 1 tsp cumin
- 14 large jalapeños
- ½ tsp pepper
- 1 cup pepper jack cheese, grated
- 2 tsp pit boss hickory bacon rub
- ½ tsp salt

Directions:

1. Fire up your Pit Boss and preheat to 400° F. If using a gas or charcoal grill, set it for medium-high heat.
2. In a food processor, combine the brisket, Hickory Bacon, cumin, salt, pepper, pepper jack and cream cheese. Pulse several times until well combined. Transfer to a bowl and place into refrigerator to chill while preparing jalapeños.
3. Place jalapeños on a sheet tray. Cut each in half lengthwise and remove the seeds and rib with a spoon or by hand, then discard. Note: we recommend using gloves when handling jalapenos, as the seeds can be very hot.
4. Fill each jalapeño half with cream cheese mixture until full, then place other jalapeño half on top. Wrap each jalapeño with a slice of bacon, then skewer crosswise with toothpicks.
5. Place a mesh, metal pan on grill grate and transfer jalapeños to pan. Cover grill and cook for 35 minutes.
6. Open grill and baste jalapeños generously with BBQ sauce, close grill and continue to cook another 5 minutes.
7. Remove from grill and serve hot.

Peppered Spicy Beef Jerky

Servings: 4-6
Cooking Time: 240 Minutes
Ingredients:

- 1 12 Oz Bottle Dark Beer
- 1/4 Cup Brown Sugar
- 2 Tbsp Coarse Black Pepper
- 4 Tbsp Garlic Salt
- 2 Tbsp Hot Sauce
- 2 Tablespoons, Divided Pit Boss Sweet Heat Rub
- 1 Tablespoon Quick Curing Salt
- 1 Cup Soy Sauce
- 2 Pounds Trimmed Flank Steak
- ¼ Worcestershire Sauce

Directions:

1. When you are ready to smoke your jerky, remove the beef from the marinade and discard the marinade.
2. Fire up your Pit Boss Smoker and set the temperature to 200°F. If using a sawdust or charcoal smoker, set it up for medium low heat.
3. Arrange the meat in a single layer directly on the smoker grate. Smoke the beef for 4-5 hours, or until the jerky is dry but still chewy and still bends somewhat.
4. Remove the jerky from the grill with tongs and transfer to a resealable plastic bag while still warm. Let the jerky rest for 1 hour at room temperature.
5. Squeeze any air out of the resealable plastic bag and refrigerate the jerky. It will keep for several weeks. Enjoy!

Bacon Wrapped Steaks

Servings: 4
Cooking Time: 15 Minutes
Ingredients:

- 1/2 Teaspoon Black Pepper
- 3 Tablespoons/ Small Chunks Butter, Unsalted Melted
- 3 1/2 Teaspoons Chives, Chopped
- 12 Large Peeled Garlic, Cloves
- 1/4 Cup Olive Oil
- Salt, Kosher

- 4 (6 - To 7 - Ounce) 1 Inch Thick Steak, Beef
- 1/2 Teaspoon Dried Thyme, Fresh Sprigs

Directions:

1. Fire up your Pit Boss Grill and turn heat to the HIGH setting. Make sure the Flame Broiler Plate is open.
2. While your grill is heating up, mix the melted butter, olive oil, kosher salt, pepper, garlic, chives, and thyme into a bowl.
3. Wrap the bacon around the sides of the steaks and hold in place with a toothpick.
4. Baste the top and bottom of the steaks with the mix using a basting brush.
5. Place the steaks on the grill and brown for 5 minutes on each side.
6. Remove steaks once internal temperature has reached the level of desired doneness.
7. Rare = 120°F
8. Medium Rare: 130°F
9. Medium: 140°F
10. Well Done: 160°F
11. After removing the steaks, let them rest for at least 5 minutes.

Bossin' Beer Can Burger Chili

Servings: 6
Cooking Time: 40 Minutes
Ingredients:

- 1 Cup Beer, Any Brand
- 1 Can Chili Beans
- 2 Tablespoons Chili Powder
- 1/2 Teaspoon Cumin
- 1 Can Green Chiles, Drained
- 1 Lb Ground Chuck
- 1 Can Kidney Beans, Drained And Rinsed
- 1 Small Onion, Diced
- 1 Tablespoon Pit Boss Hickory Bacon Seasoning
- 1 Large Can Tomato Sauce
- 1 Can Fire Roasted Tomatoes

Directions:

1. In a pan on a stove top, sauté the diced onions in butter or oil until light yellow. Add in ground chuck and sprinkle with a teaspoon of salt and pepper. Cook until ground chuck is light brown.
2. In a disposable aluminum pan, mix all the ingredients (including the sautéed ground chuck and onions) thoroughly. Cover tightly with aluminum foil.
3. Place the aluminum pan on the grill for 30-40 minutes, or until the chili has thickened and is bubbling. Remove from the grill and serve.

Cheddar Stuffed Burgers

Servings: 12
Cooking Time: 30 Minutes
Ingredients:

- Bacon Cheddar Burger Seasoning
- 3/4 Cup Bacon, Chopped
- 3 Lbs Beef, Ground
- 1 Jalapeno, Chopped
- Pepper
- 1/2 Cup Ranch Dressing
- Salt
- 1 1/2 Cups Shredded Cheddar Cheese

Directions:

1. Set your Pit Boss grill to 350°F
2. In a small bowl, combine cheese, bacon, jalapeno and ranch dressing.
3. In a clean, large bowl, combine ground beef with enough salt and pepper to taste.
4. Form meat into patties and place on a pan. A good rule of thumb is for each patty to be about the size of the palm of your hand.
5. Using a clean glass, press into each patty, leaving the imprint of the bottom of the glass in the patty. Stuff the filling into the indent. Grill for 25 minutes or until the ground beef reaches an internal temperature of 160°F. Serve hot.

Grilled Tri Tip With Cajun Butter

Servings: 2
Cooking Time: 20 Minutes
Ingredients:

- 4 Tablespoons Beef & Brisket Rub
- 1/3 Cup Brown Sugar
- 1 Stick Unsalted Softened Butter
- 1/2 Tsp Cayenne Pepper
- 1 Garlic Clove, Minced
- 2 Tablespoons Olive Oil
- Juice From 1 Orange
- 1 Tbsp Paprika, Powder
- 1/3 Cup Soy Sauce
- 3 - 4 Pounds Trimmed Tri Tip Roast
- 2 Tablespoons Worcestershire Sauce

Directions:

1. Add the brown sugar, orange juice, Worcestershire sauce, minced garlic and soy sauce to a resealable plastic bag. Add the tri tip to the bag, seal it, and massage the meat to help coat it evenly with the marinade. Place the bag in the refrigerator and allow the tri tip to marinate for 2 hours.
2. Remove the bag from the refrigerator and drain the marinade. Remove the steak from the bag and pat dry with paper towels.
3. In a small mixing bowl, combine the softened butter with 2 tablespoons of Beef & Brisket Seasoning, paprika, and cayenne. Mix the butter until well combined. Set aside.
4. Rub the tri tip down with the olive oil and season generously with the remaining Beef & Brisket Seasoning.
5. Fire up your Pit Boss Grill and set the temperature to 450°F. If you're using a gas or charcoal grill, set it up for high heat. Insert a temperature probe into the thickest part of the steak and place it on the grill. Sear the tri tip on the grill for 3-5 minutes, then flip it and sear for another 3-5 minutes.
6. Turn the temperature down to 250°F, then grill the tri tip for 15 more minutes until the internal temperature reaches 135°F.

Reverse Seared Picanha Steak

Servings: 4
Cooking Time:120 Mins
Ingredients:

- olive oil
- 3 lbs picanha steak, top sirloin cap, fat cap removed
- tt pit boss chop house steak rub

Directions:

1. Fire up your Pit Boss Platinum Series KC Combo and preheat to 225°F. If using a gas or charcoal grill, set it up for low, indirect heat.
2. Generously season both sides of steak with Chop House, insert temperature probe, and place steak directly on the grill grate.
3. Cover grill and cook 1 ½ to 2 hours, or until internal temperature reads 125°F to 130°F.
4. Remove steak from grill, then preheat KC Combo griddle to medium-high flame. Heat olive oil on the griddle, then sear steak 2 minutes per side on all sides.
5. Remove steak from the griddle, and allow to rest on a cutting board for 10 minutes. Slice steak, against the grain, and serve warm.

Beef Short Rib Burger

Servings: 4
Cooking Time: 30 Minutes
Ingredients:

- 1/4 Cup Barbecue Sauce
- 4 Cheddar Cheese, Slices
- 4 Eggs
- 1 Pound Ground Chuck

- 1/2 Tablespoon Olive Oil
- 1 Tablespoon Pit Boss Beef And Brisket Rub
- 1/2 Cup Cooked Shredded Beef Rib(S)

Directions:

1. Start up your Pit Boss. Then, set the temperature to 350°F.
2. In a large bowl, mix the ground chuck and, Beef and Brisket Rub until evenly combined. Shape into patties.
3. Grill the patties for 7-10 minutes, flipping halfway and topping with a slice of cheddar cheese. When the burgers are to the desired degree of doneness, remove from the grill and set aside.
4. In a small bowl, mix the short rib and barbecue sauce.
5. In a small frying pan, heat the olive oil over medium-low heat and fry the eggs until the white is firm and the yolk is runny.
6. Assemble the burgers: top each bun with a burger patty, a spoonful of the short rib mixture, and a fried egg. Serve and enjoy

Kansas City Brisket Burger

Servings: 4
Cooking Time: 30 Minutes
Ingredients:

- 1/2 Cup Barbecue Sauce
- 4 Brioche Burger Buns
- 4 Slices Brisket
- 1 Lbs Ground Beef
- 8 Onion Rings
- 4 Tablespoons Pit Boss Sweet Rib Rub
- 4 Slices Smoked Guoda Cheese, Sliced

Directions:

1. In a large bowl, sprinkle the Pit Boss Sweet Rib Rub over the ground beef and mix well to combine. Shape the ground beef into 4 patties and set aside.

2. Preheat your Pit Boss Grill to 350°F. Grill your burgers for 8-10 minutes, or until desired degree of doneness.
3. Halfway through cooking, top each burger patty with a slice of smoked gouda cheese.
4. Remove the burgers from the grill and assemble the burgers. Place each burger on a bun and top with 2 tablespoons of barbecue sauce, 2 onion rings and a slice of brisket, then serve and enjoy!

Brisket Style Tri Tip

Servings: 4
Cooking Time: 300 Mins
Ingredients:

- bbq sauce
- dill pickles
- jalapeño
- to taste, java chophouse seasoning
- 2 tbsp mustard
- onion, sliced & minced
- 2 lbs tri tip steak

Directions:

1. Fire up your Pit Boss and with the lid open, set your temperature to SMOKE mode.
2. Once the fire is lit, preheat to 225° F. If using a gas or charcoal grill, set it up for low, indirect heat.
3. Rub the mustard all over the tri tip, then season with Java Chophouse.
4. Place the tri tip directly on the grill grates and smoke until the internal temperature reaches 165° F (about 2 1/2 hours).
5. Remove the tri tip from the grill and wrap it in Pit Boss butcher paper. Return the tri tip to the grill and continue to smoke until the internal temperature reaches 200° F (an additional 2 ½ to 3 hours).
6. Remove the tri tip from the grill, and rest for 30 minutes. Slice thin and serve with pickles, jalapeño, onion, and BBQ sauce, if desired.

Philly Cheesesteak Burger

Servings: 4
Cooking Time: 30 Minutes
Ingredients:

- 4 Burger Buns
- 1 Green Bell Pepper, Sliced
- 1 Pound Ground Beef
- 1 Tablespoon Olive Oil
- 1 Tablespoon Pit Boss Chop House Steak Seasoning
- 4 Provolone Cheese, Sliced

Directions:

1. In a large bowl, mix the ground beef and Pit Boss Chop House Steal seasoning together until well combined. Form into patties. Preheat your Pit Boss grill to 350°F and grill for 5-7 minutes, flipping halfway through. Once you flip the burgers, top with a slice of provolone cheese.
2. Once the burgers have cooked to your desired degree of doneness, remove from the grill and set aside.
3. For the pepper and onion: in a sauté pan over medium heat, heat the olive oil until it shimmers, then add the onion and pepper. Cook until the pepper and onion are soft and start to caramelize and develop a little char, about 15 minutes.

Leftover Brisket Tostadas With Beans & Cheese

Servings: 4
Cooking Time: 30 Minutes
Ingredients:

- 2 Cups Leftover Chopped Brisket
- Lime, Wedges
- Pickled Jalapeno
- 1 Cup Refried Beans
- ½ Cup Salsa
- 8 Tostada Shells
- ½ Cup Shredded Cheddar Cheese

Directions:

1. Start up your Pit Boss. Once it's fired up, set the temperature to 300°F.
2. Assemble the tostadas: smear a tostada shell with refried beans and top with cheese and brisket. Repeat with a second shell and place on top of the first.
3. Grill the tostadas for 5-10 minutes, or until everything is warmed through and the cheese is melty. Remove from the grill.
4. Top the tostadas with tomatoes, cilantro, pickled jalapenos, etc and serve immediately!

Java Chophouse Steak Tips With Mashed Potatoes

Servings: 4-6
Cooking Time: 60 Minutes
Ingredients:

- 1 Cup Beef Broth
- 1 Stick (Room Temperature) Butter, Unsalted
- 2 Tablespoon Flour, All-Purpose
- 1 Tablespoon Pit Boss Java Chophouse Seasoning
- 4 Tablespoon Pit Boss Java Chophouse Seasoning, Divided
- 2 Pounds Medium Russet Potatoes, Peele And Cut (Large Chunks)
- 2 Pounds Strip Sirloin
- 1/2 To 1 Cup Whole Milk, Warm

Directions:

1. For the mashed potatoes: add the potatoe to a large pot and add enough cold water to cover the potatoes. Bring to a simmer over medium heat until the potatoes are tender enough to be pierced with a fork, about 40 minutes. Drain the potatoes.
2. Add the potatoes to a large mixing bowl. Add the butter, 1 tablespoon of Java Chop House and ½ cup of warm milk. Mash until smooth and lump free. If potatoes are too thick, add more milk, a tablespoon at a time, until you reach your desired consistency.

3. For the steak tips: preheat your Pit Boss grill to 350°F. Season the steaks generously on both sides with 2 tablespoons of Java Chop House seasoning and grill for 8-10 minutes per side. When steaks are done, remove from grill, allow to rest for 15 minutes, then cut into chunks.

4. While the steak is resting, add the butter to a small saucepan over low heat. Once the butter is melted, whisk in the flour and cook for 2 minutes until the flour smells toasted. Slowly whisk in the beef broth and remaining 2 tablespoons of Java Chop H ouse seasoning and cook the gravy over low heat until thickened. Remove from heat and toss the steak tips in the gravy.

5. Serve steak tips over mashed potatoes. Enjoy!

Cowgirl Steak & Eggs On The Griddle

Servings: 2
Cooking Time:15 Mins
Ingredients:

- , 1 lbs cowgirl ribeye steak
- 4 eggs
- 1/2 jalapeno pepper, minced
- 1 tbsp olive oil
- tt pit boss chop house steak rub
- 1 scallion, sliced thin
- 1 lb yukon gold potatoes

Directions:

1. Fire up your Pit Boss griddle and preheat to medium-high flame.

2. Season steaks generously with Pit Boss Chop House Rub. Drizzle olive oil on the hot skillet, then sear steaks for 5 to 7 minutes per side, depending on thickness, for medium-rare.

3. After the final sear, quickly sear edges, then add a tablespoon or two of butter, and quickly baste the steaks, turning with tongs. Transfer steaks to a cutting board, to rest for 5 minutes.

4. Meanwhile, halve the par-boiled potatoes. Season with more Chop House Rub.

5. While steaks are resting, sear potatoes in 1 tablespoon of butter, 2 minutes per side. Add jalapeño and scallions at the end, then remove from the griddle.

6. After the first turn of the potatoes, add remaining butter and a drizzle of olive oil in the middle of the griddle. Crack 4 eggs on top. Cook for 2 minutes, or until the white is opaque, but yolk remains runny.

7. Plate sliced steak with 2 sunny-side-up eggs and potatoes.

Tomahawk Prime Rib

Servings: 10 - 12
Cooking Time: 240 Minutes
Ingredients:

- 1 Stick Of Butter
- 3/4 Cup Extra-Virgin Olive Oil
- 5 Garlic, Cloves
- Pit Boss Sweet Heat Rub
- 2 Tablespoon Rosemary, Fresh
- Tomahawk Prime Rib
- 2 Cups White Wine
- 1 Cup Worcestershire Sauce

Directions:

1. Cook the baste. Melt 1 stick of butter in saucepan with 2 cloves garlic. Add 2 cups white wine of your choice with enough Worcestershire Sauce to make a brown iced tea color.

2. Start your Pit Boss on SMOKE Mode with the lid open. Let the pellets catch fire in the burn pot, close the lid, and heat your grill to 250°F.

3. Apply the baste all over the prime rib and smoke at 250°F until it reaches an internal temp of 120°F.

4. Apply the dry rub – Blend: 2-3 cloves of garlic, 2 tbsp fresh rosemary, ½ cup Extra Virgin Olive Oil, ¼ cup of Pit Boss Sweet

Heat Rub. Pour over prime rib and rub all over.

5. Raise grill temp to 425°F, open the Flame Broiler Plate and sear until the meat reaches an internal temperature of 125°F-135°F.

Classic Smoked Brisket

Servings: 8
Cooking Time: 480 Minutes
Ingredients:

- 1 - 12-15 Lbs Beef, Brisket
- Pit Boss Beef And Brisket Rub

Directions:

1. Turn your Pit Boss to smoke mode, let the fire catch and then set your grill to 225°F.
2. While your grill is heating up, trim your brisket of excess fat (you'll want to leave about ¼ of an inch of fat so the meat stays moist during the long cooking process) , and season with your favorite rub - whatever floats your boat! Place your brisket on the grates of the grill, fat side up. Let it smoke for about 8 - 10 hours, or until the internal temperature reaches 190°F.
3. Wrap in pink butcher paper and then wrap that in a towel. Let it rest in the cooler for up to an hour so the juices can sit.
4. Slice against the grain and enjoy!

Breakfast Cheeseburger

Servings: 2
Cooking Time: 10 Minutes
Ingredients:

- 4 Bacon, Strip
- 6 Ounce Lean Beef, Ground
- 2 Burger Buns
- 2 Cheese, Sliced
- 2 Egg
- Pepper
- Salt

Directions:

1. Start your Grill on "smoke" with the lid open until a fire is established in the burn pot (3-7 minutes). Preheat to 400°F.
2. Take the ground beef and divide it into two thin patties. Brush the grate with oil, then add the patties and grill them on about 2-5 minutes on each side, or until the desired doneness, pressing down to get a good sear.
3. Remove the burgers from the grill, then build your burger. Starting with the bottom bun or bread slice, add the patty, then a slice of American cheese, top with bacon, hash browns, an egg over easy, and finish with the top bun or bread slice. Now it's ready to serve!

Bbq Brisket Queso

Servings: 6
Cooking Time: 15 Minutes
Ingredients:

- ½ Cup Barbecue Sauce
- 1 Cup Brisket, Pulled
- 2 Tablespoons Butter
- 1 Pound American Or Velveeta Cheese, Cubed
- 1 Cup Green Chili, Chopped
- 1 Cup Heavy Cream
- Serving Pickled Jalapeno
- Serving Salsa
- 1 Cup Tomato, Diced
- Serving Tortilla Chip
- ½ Of One Finely Diced White Onions

Directions:

1. Fire up your Pit Boss and set the temperature to 300°F. If you're using gas or charcoal, set your grill for medium low, indirect heat.
2. Let the grilling skillet heat up on the grill. Then, add the 2 tablespoons of butter and finely diced onion and sauté the onions until they are soft and translucent.

3. Next, pour in the heavy cream and bring it to a simmer. Once the cream is simmering, add the cubed cheese, diced tomatoes, and chopped green chilis. Make sure to stir the mixture consistently until the cheese is completely melted.

4. In a separate bowl, combine the brisket with the barbecue sauce and toss until the brisket is fully covered.

5. When your queso is ready, pour it into a serving bowl and top with the brisket, salsa, and jalapenos. You can even add fresh cilantro as a garnish.

6. Serve the queso with tortilla chips while it's hot and fresh and enjoy.

alapeno Burgers With Bacon nd Pepper Jack Cheese

ervings: 4
ooking Time: 30 Minutes
ngredients:

- 4 Slices, Raw Bacon
- 1/2 Cup Prepared Barbecue Sauce
- 1 Pound Ground Beef
- Hickory Bacon Seasoning, Plus More For Sprinkling
- 2 Thinly Sliced Jalapeno Peppers
- 1/2 Cup Olive Oil
- 4 Onion Burger Buns
- Onion, Crispy
- 4 Pepper Jack Cheese, Sliced

Directions:

1. Fire up your Pit Boss and set the temperature to 350°F. If using a gas or charcoal grill, set it up for medium high heat.

2. Make the burgers: in a large bowl, mix together the ground beef and Hickory Bacon seasoning until the seasoning is well incorporated. Use the Burger Press to make burger patties. Repeat until all the ground beef is gone.

3. In a small bowl, toss the sliced raw jalapenos with the olive oil and place them in the vegetable grill basket. Grill the jalapenos, stirring occasionally, until soft and charred in some spots. Remove from the grill and set aside.

4. Place the bacon on the vegetable grill basket and grill for 5-7 minutes, or until the bacon is crispy and brown. Remove from the grill and set aside.

5. Grill the burgers: place the burger patties on the grill and, if desired, sprinkle more Hickory Bacon seasoning on the patties. Grill the burgers for 5 minutes on one side, then flip and top with a slice of pepper jack cheese and grill for another 5-7 minutes, or until the internal temperature of the burgers is 135-140°F.

6. Remove the burgers from the grill and place on an onion bun. Top with the bacon, grilled jalapenos, crisped onions, and a spoonful of barbecue sauce.

Chili Bratwurst

Servings: 4
Cooking Time: 45 Minutes
Ingredients:

- 1 Chopped Chipotle In Adobo
- 3 - 4 Cans Of Beer, Any Brand
- 4 Bratwursts, Raw
- 4 Bratwurst Buns
- ½ Cup Prepared Nacho Cheese Sauce
- 1 Cup Chili, Prepared
- Caramelized Onions
- Sweet Rib Rub

Directions:

1. Set up your Pit Boss. Once it's fired up, set the temperature to 350°F. If you're using charcoal or gas, set the temperature to medium high.

2. Place a pot filled with beer, Sweet Rib Rub, caramelized onions and raw brats. Place on grill and par-boil for 20 minutes.

3. Grill the brats for 7-10 minutes, or until internal temperature of the brats is 160°F. Remove the brats from the grill and allow them to rest for 5 minutes.
4. While the brats rest, place the chili in a sauce pan, and place the sauce pan on the grill. Heat the chili all the way through.
5. In a separate sauce pan, add the nacho cheese to the pan, add adobo chili peppers and a shake of Sweet Rib Rub. Place the saucepan on the grill and heat until warm all the way through.
6. Assemble the brats: place a brat in a bun, then top with a spoonful of chili and a spoonful of nacho cheese. Serve immediately.

CHICKEN RECIPES

Bbq Chicken Stuffed Bell Peppers

Servings: 4
Cooking Time: 15 Minutes
Ingredients:

- ½ Cup Barbecue Sauce
- 4 Bell Pepper
- ½ Cup Cheddar Cheese, Shredded
- 2 Cups Leftover Chicken, Chopped
- 2 Tablespoons Champion Chicken Seasoning

Directions:

1. Wash and slice the bell peppers in half, long ways. Deseed them and set aside.
2. Preheat your Pit Boss. Once it's fired up, set the temperature to 350°F.
3. In a large bowl, mix together the cheese, chicken, Champion Chicken Seasoning, and barbecue sauce, then stuff inside the pepper halves.
4. Grill the peppers for 7-10 minutes or until the peppers are softened and the filling is heated through and melted. Remove from the grill and serve.

Bourbon Breaded Chicken And Waffles

Servings: 8
Cooking Time: 30 Minutes
Ingredients:

- 1 Shot Of Bourbon
- 3 Cups Bread Crumbs
- 4 Horizontally Half Sliced Boneless, Skinless Chicken Breast
- Butter Flavored Cooking Spray
- 3 Eggs
- 1 Tsp Garlic Powder
- 1 Tsp Paprika, Powder
- Red Velvet Cake Mix
- 16 Oz. Reduced Fat Sour Cream

- Sweet Rib Rub
- ¼ Cup Vegetable Oil
- 1 ¼ Cup Water
- 1 Tbsp Worcestershire Sauce

Directions:

1. Fire up your Pit Boss and set the temperature to 350°F. If you're using a gas or charcoal grill, set up the grill for medium heat.
2. In a large bowl, combine the sour cream, bourbon, Worcestershire sauce, paprika, garlic powder, and Sweet Rib Rub seasoning. Add the chicken, turn the chicken breasts to coat, and cover the bowl. Refrigerate for 4-12 hrs.
3. Remove the chicken from the refrigerator and drain the marinade from the chicken. Mix together 3 cups bread crumbs and 2 tbsp Sweet Rib Rub. Mix the coating together and bread the chicken breasts.
4. Moisten a paper towel with cooking oil and using a pair of tongs, lightly grease the grill rack.
5. Grill or smoke until the internal temperature of the chicken reaches 170°F and the chicken is crispy and golden brown.
6. While the chicken is cooking, mix the eggs, vegetable oil, water, and red velvet cake mix in a bowl with the electric mixer.
7. Add the mix into the waffle iron and cook. Make as many waffles as the mix allows.
8. On a plate, place the cooked chicken on top of the waffles and top with maple syrup or honey.

Whole Smoked Chicken With Honey Glaze

Servings: 4
Cooking Time: 40 Minutes
Ingredients:

- 1 Tablespoon Honey
- 1 ½ Lemon

- 4 Tablespoons Pit Boss Champion Chicken Seasoning
- 4 Tablespoons Unsalted Butter
- 1, 4 Pound Chicken, Giblets Removed And Patted Dry

Directions:

1. Start up your Pit Boss Smoker. Once it's fired up, set the temperature to 225°F.
2. In a small saucepan, melt together the butter and honey over low heat. Squeeze ½ lemon into the honey mixture and remove from the heat.
3. Smoke the chicken, skin side down until the chicken is lightly browned and the skin releases from the grate without ripping, about 6-8 minutes.
4. Turn the chicken over and baste with the honey butter mixture.
5. Continue to smoke the chicken, basting every 45 minutes, until the thickest part of the chicken reaches 160°F.

Buffalo Ranch Chicken Wings

Servings: 4
Cooking Time: 20 Minutes
Ingredients:

- 1 1/2 Tbsp Apple Cider Vinegar
- 1/2 Cup Butter, Unsalted, Cubed
- 1/4 Tsp Cayenne Pepper
- 3 Lbs Chicken Wings, Split
- 2 Tsp Chives, Minced (Garnish)
- 1/8 Tsp Garlic, Granulated
- 2/3 Cup Hot Pepper Sauce
- 1 Tbsp Ranch Seasoning
- To Taste, Sweet Heat Rub
- 1/2 Tsp Sweet Heat Rub (For Sauce)
- 1/4 Tsp Worcestershire Sauce

Directions:

1. Fire up your Pit Boss pellet grill on SMOKE mode and let it run with lid open for 10 minutes then preheat to 425° F. If

using a gas or charcoal grill, set it up for medium-high heat.

2. Place chicken wings in a large mixing bowl. Season with Sweet Heat.
3. Prepare sauce: Set a small cast iron pan or saucepan on the grill. Add the hot pepper sauce, apple cider vinegar, Worcestershire sauce, Sweet Heat, cayenne, and granulated garlic to the skillet, and whisk to combine. When the sauce begins to bubble, remove the skillet from the grill and whisk in butter. Transfer the sauce to a mason jar.
4. Combine 1 cup of the buffalo sauce with ranch seasoning. Set aside.
5. Place wings on the grill and cook for 20 minutes, flipping and rotating every 3 to 5 minutes.
6. Remove wings from the grill when an internal temperature of 165° F is reached. Transfer to a mixing bowl, then pour sauce over. Toss to evenly coat. Garnish with fresh chives and serve warm.

Chicken Lollipops With Sticky Asian Sauce

Servings: 3
Cooking Time: 45 Minutes
Ingredients:

- To Taste, Blackened Sriracha Rub Seasoning
- 1/4 Cup Brown Sugar
- 3 Lbs Chicken Drumsticks
- 2 Garlic Cloves, Minced
- 2 Tbsp Honey
- 1" Knob Of Ginger Root, Grated
- 2 Tsp Sesame Oil
- For Garnish, Sliced Scallions
- 3 Tbsp Sweet Chili Sauce
- 1/4 Cup Tamari
- For Garnish, Toasted Sesame Seeds
- 2 Tsp Vegetable Oil

1. Prepare lollipops: Use a sharp knife coupled with kitchen shears to cut around the leg, just below the knuckle, then tear/clip off. Cut out loose skin, tendons, and clip the small bone against the leg, then push the meat down. Transfer to a sheet tray while repeating with remaining chicken legs. Season with Blackened Sriracha.
2. Fire up your Pit Boss pellet grill on SMOKE mode and let it run with lid open for 10 minutes then preheat to 350° F. If using a gas or charcoal grill, set it up for medium heat.
3. Place the chicken lollipops on the grill, over indirect heat and cook for 25 to 30 minutes, flipping and rotating occasionally, until an internal temperature of 165° F is reached.
4. Remove from the grill and rest for 10 minutes.
5. While lollipops are resting, prepare the sauce: Place a small cast iron skillet on the grill. Add sesame oil, vegetable oil, honey, sweet chili sauce, brown sugar, tamari, ginger, and garlic. Whisk to combine, then bring to a simmer. Simmer for 5 minutes until sauce thickens and sugar is dissolved.
6. Remove skillet from the grill, cool for 5 minutes, then roll each lollipop in the sauce. Transfer to a platter, and garnish with scallions and toasted sesame seeds. Serve warm.

Grilled Chicken Kabobs

Servings: 6
Cooking Time: 15 Minutes
Ingredients:

- 3 (Cut Into 1 Inch Cubes) Chicken Breast, Raw
- 2 Cloves Garlic, Minced
- 2 Tablespoons Honey
- 1 Pound Of Button (Destemmed And Cut In Half) Mushroom
- 1/2 Cup Olive Oil
- 1 Red (Cut Into Quarters And Seperated) Onion
- 1 Green (Cut Into Large Chunks) Bell Pepper
- 2 Tablespoons Pit Boss Competition Smoked Seasoning
- 2 Tablespoons Soy Sauce

Directions:

1. To make the marinade: In a large bowl, combine the olive oil, soy sauce, honey, garlic and Competition Smoked. Add the chicken and mix well. When the chicken is covered completely, allow it to marinate for 2-12 hours.
2. In a large, shallow baking dish, soak the kabob skewers for a minimum of 2 hours and up to 12 hours.
3. Once the chicken has finished marinating and the skewers are finished soaking, drain the water from the skewers and remove the chicken from the marinade.
4. Start your Pit Boss on "smoke". Once it's fired up, set the temperature to 350°F.
5. Thread a piece of chicken, followed by a piece of pepper, mushroom, and onion. Repeat until the skewers are full.
6. Grill the kabobs for 5 minutes on one side, then flip and grill for 5 more minutes or until the chicken reaches an internal temperature of 180°F. Remove from the grill and serve.

Lemon Garlic Parmesan Chicken Wings

Servings: 4 -8
Cooking Time: 30 Minutes
Ingredients:

- 2 Tablespoons Unsalted Butter, Melted
- 2 Lbs Chicken Wings, Trimmed And Patted Dry

- 3 Cloves Garlic, Minced
- Juice Of 1 Lemon
- 2 Tablespoons Mustard, Dijon
- ¼ Cup Olive Oil
- ¼ Cup Shredded Parmesan Cheese
- 2 Tablespoons Parsley, Chopped
- 2 Tablespoons Champion Chicken Seasoning

Directions:

1. Set up your Pit Boss Grill. Once it's fired up, set the temperature to 350°F. If you are using a charcoal or gas grill, set the temperature to medium high heat.
2. In a large resealable bag, combine the olive oil, minced garlic, lemon zest, lemon juice, Dijon mustard, Champion Chicken Seasoning, and chopped parsley. Seal the resealable bag and give it a good shake to mix the ingredients.
3. Once the chicken has finished marinating, remove the chicken from the marinade and drain. Place the chicken wings on the wing rack.
4. Place the wing rack on the grill and insert a temperature probe into the thickest part of one of the wings. Grill the wings for 5 minutes, then rotate, and grill for another 5-10 minutes, or until the internal temperature of the wings reaches 165°F.
5. Toss the wings in the large bowl with the melted butter and shredded Parmesan until well coated. Serve immediately.

Jerk Chicken Wings

Servings: 0
Cooking Time: 0 Minutes

Ingredients:

- 1 Tsp Allspice, Ground
- 3 Lbs Chicken Wings, Split
- 1/2 Tsp Cinnamon, Ground
- 4 Garlic Cloves, Smashed
- 2 Tsp Ginger, Grated
- 1 Habanero Pepper, Chopped
- 2 Tbsp Honey
- 2 Tbsp Lemon Juice
- 1/3 Cup Lime Juice
- 1/2 Tsp Nutmeg, Ground
- 1/2 Cup Olive Oil
- 1/4 Cup Poblano Pepper, Chopped
- 1 Tbsp Tamari
- 2 Tsp Thyme, Dried
- 1/2 Cup Yellow Onion, Chopped

Directions:

1. Add chicken to a large resealable plastic bag.
2. In the bowl of a food processor, add the garlic, onion, ginger, peppers, tamari, honey, lime juice, lemon juice, thyme, allspice, cinnamon, nutmeg, and oil. Process on low for 1 minute, then transfer marinade to the bag. Seal the bag and place in the refrigerator for at least 2 hours, up to overnight.
3. Fire up your Pit Boss pellet grill on SMOKE mode and let it run with lid open for 10 minutes then preheat to 425° F. If using a gas or charcoal grill, set it up for medium-high heat.
4. Remove wings from the marinade, and discard remaining marinade. Place wings on the grill and cook for 15 to 20 minutes, flipping every 5 minutes, until an internal temperature of 165 F is reached.
5. Remove wings from the grill and serve warm.

Grilled Chicken Burrito Bowls

Servings: 4

Cooking Time: 20 Minutes

Ingredients:

- 1 Avocado
- 1 Can Black Beans, Rinsed And Drained
- 1 ½ Pounds Boneless Skinless Chicken Strips
- 1 Tablespoon Cilantro, Chopped
- 1 Can Corn Kernels, Drained
- Juice From 1 Lime
- ½ Lime Lime Juice
- 1 ½ Cups Long Grain White Rice
- 2 Tablespoons Olive Oil
- 2 Tablespoons Pit Boss Sweet Heat Rub
- ¼ Cup Salsa
- 1 Teaspoon Salt
- ½ Cup Shredded Mexican Blend Cheese
- ¼ Cup Sour Cream

Directions:

1. Fire up your Pit Boss and set the temperature to 350°F. If using a gas or charcoal grill, set it up for medium heat.
2. Place the rice in a fine mesh sieve and rinse under cold water for 2-5 minutes, or until the water runs clear. Add the rice to a pot with 2 cups of water and 1 teaspoon of salt and bring to a boil on the stove top. Once the rice boils, drop the temperature to a simmer, place the pot lid on top securely, and let the rice cook for 20-25 minutes.
3. Once the time is up, remove the rice from the heat, and allow it to steam with the lid on for a further 10 minutes. Remove the lid from the rice, add the lime juice and cilantro, and fluff the rice with a fork. Set aside.
4. Grill the chicken for 5-7 minutes, or until the chicken reaches an internal temperature of 165°F and is golden and charred in some spots. Remove the chicken from the grill and allow it to rest

for 5 minutes before slicing into bite sized pieces.

5. To assemble the burrito bowls: place a large scoop of cilantro lime rice into a bowl. Top with slices of grilled chicken, a scoop of black beans, a scoop of corn, salsa, cheese, sour cream, and avocado. Serve immediately.

Asian Bbq Wings

Servings: 6

Cooking Time: 60 Minutes

Ingredients:

- 2 Lbs Chicken, Wing
- 1 Tsp Garlic, Minced
- 1 Tsp Ginger, Fresh
- 1 Tsp Chopped Green Onion
- 1/2 Cup Hoisin Sauce
- 1 Tsp Honey
- 2 Tsp Rice Vinegar
- 2 Tsp Sesame Oil
- 1 Tsp Sesame Seeds
- 1 Tsp Soy Sauce
- 1 Cup Water, Boiling

Directions:

1. Add all ingredients except wings and sesame seeds to a mixing bowl and whisk to incorporate. Add wings to a resealable plastic bag and pour marinade over. Allow marinating for at least 2 hours up to overnight. Remove wings from bag, reserving marinade.
2. Preheat grill to 300°F. Place wings in a grilling basket and cook for 1 hour or until they reach an internal temperature of 165°F.
3. While wings are cooking, pour reserved marinade into a small saucepan and add rice wine vinegar. Over high heat, bring to a boil while whisking often, and reduce by 1/3, or about 10 minutes. Set aside.
4. Brush wings with reduced sauce and allow to cook for 5-10 more minutes or until

glaze has set. Remove from smoker, sprinkle with sesame seeds, allow to rest for 5 minutes, and serve.

Garlic Sriracha Chicken Wings

Servings: 6-8
Cooking Time: 160 Minutes
Ingredients:
- 1 Cup Buffalo Sauce
- 6 Lbs Chicken Wings
- 2 Tbsp Garlic Powder
- 1 Tsp Pepper
- Divided By 2 Tbsp And ½ Tbsp Pit Boss Sweet Heat Rub
- 1 Tsp Salt
- ⅓ Cup, Divided Sriracha Sauce

Directions:
1. In a non-stick sauce pot, add the remaining Sriracha and buffalo sauce. Stir to combine and set aside.
2. Fire up your Pit Boss and preheat to 250° F. If using a gas or charcoal grill, set it to low heat with indirect heat. Place marinated wings directly on grill grate and cook (covered) for 1 hour 15 minutes.
3. Flip wings and baste each piece with Sriracha sauce. Season with additional Pit Boss Sweet Heat Rub, cover, and continue to grill for an additional 1 hour 15 minutes.
4. Remove wings from grill and place on sheet tray. Baste with additional sauce, then open Sear Slide and return wings to the grill. Grill for 3-5 minutes, rotating often, until wings begin to char lightly.
5. Transfer wings to a serving tray, baste with remaining sauce and serve!

Grilled Parmesan Garlic Chicken Wings

Servings: 4
Cooking Time: 25 Minutes
Ingredients:

- 4 Tbsp Butter
- 4 Lbs Chicken Wings, Trimmed And Patted Dry
- 4 Garlic Cloves, Chopped
- 2 Tbsp Olive Oil
- 1/2 Cup Parmesan Cheese, Grated
- 2 Tbsp Parsley, Chopped
- Tt Pit Boss Champion Chicken Seasoning

Directions:
1. Lay chicken wings out on a sheet tray, blot with paper towel, then season with Champion Chicken.
2. Fire up your Pit Boss grill and preheat to 400°F. If using a gas or charcoal grill, set it up for medium-high heat.
3. Transfer wings to grill and cook for 20 to 25 minutes, turning every 5 minutes, until lightly browned. Remove wings from the grill and set on a sheet tray. Place in the smoking cabinet to keep warm while preparing the garlic butter.
4. Melt butter and olive oil in a cast iron skillet, then add garlic and simmer until fragrant. Remove from the grill.
5. Transfer chicken wings to a large bowl and pour garlic butter over the wings. Add cheese and parsley, then toss well to coat. Serve warm with additional sprinkling of parmesan cheese.

Alabama White Sauce On Crispy Chicken Quarters

Servings: 4
Cooking Time: 55 Minutes
Ingredients:

- 2 Cups Alabama White Sauce
- 1 Tbsp Champion Chicken
- 4 Chicken Leg Quarters
- 1 Tbsp Olive Oil

Directions:

1. Place chicken leg quarters on a sheet tray lined with aluminum foil. Gently pull away the skin from the chicken leg quarters, then drizzle inside and out with olive oil. Season the chicken leg quarters all over and under the skin with Champion Chicken. Let chicken sit out at room temperature for 1 hour.
2. Fire up your Pit Boss grill and preheat to 450°F with the Sear Slide open. If using a gas or charcoal grill, set it up for medium-high heat and direct heat.
3. Sear the leg quarters on all sides over direct flame until crispy and golden brown. Transfer to indirect heat and close the sear slide. Reduce temperature to 350° F and grill the chicken for 45 minutes, turning occasionally, until chicken registers an internal temperature of 165° F.
4. Remove chicken from grill and allow to rest for 10 minutes. Serve chicken hot with a generous drizzling of Alabama white sauce*.

Champion Beer Can Chicken On The Grill

Servings: 4
Cooking Time: 75 Minutes
Ingredients:

- 3 Tbsp Barbecue Sauce
- 1 Can Beer, Any Brand
- 2 Tbsp Olive Oil
- 4-6 Tbsp Pit Boss Champion Chicken Seasoning
- 1 Whole Chicken

Directions:

1. Remove the chicken from the bag and make sure all the giblets and organs are removed from inside the chicken. Rinse the bird, inside and out, then pat dry.
2. Pour out half a can of beer until you have half a can remaining. Into the can of beer, or a chicken throne, add the barbecue sauce. Set aside.
3. Brush the chicken generously with olive oil and season with Pit Boss Champion Chicken Seasoning. Let the chicken sit for at least 15 minutes with the seasoning on top.
4. Carefully slide the chicken onto the beer can or chicken throne so that the cavity fits snugly. Tuck the chicken wings behind the chicken's back.

Zesty Chile Cilantro Lime Chicken Wings

Servings: 4
Cooking Time: 20 Minutes
Ingredients:

- 1 Tsp Ancho Chili Powder
- 2 Tsp Blackened Sriracha Rub Seasoning
- 2 Lbs Chicken Wings, Split
- 2 Tbsp Cilantro, Chopped, Divided
- 1 Tsp Cumin
- 1 Lime, Zest & Juice
- 1 1/2 Tbsp Olive Oil

Directions:

1. In a medium bowl, combine 1 tablespoon of cilantro, lime juice and zest, olive oil, Blackened Sriracha, ancho chili powder, and cumin.
2. Place chicken wings in a resealable gallon bag and add cilantro mixture. Transfer to

the refrigerator and marinate for 1 hour, turning occasionally.

3. Fire up your Pit Boss Platinum Series KC Combo and set it to 350° F. If using a gas or charcoal grill, set it up for medium heat.
4. Remove chicken wings from the marinade and place on the grill over indirect heat. Grill for 15 to 18 minutes, turning and rotating every 3 to 5 minutes.
5. Remove chicken wings from the grill, garnish with remaining cilantro, and serve warm.

Chicken Cordon Bleu

Servings: 8
Cooking Time: 75 Minutes
Ingredients:
- 8 Chicken, Boneless/Skinless
- 1 Cup Mozzarella Cheese, Shredded
- Pit Boss Lemon Pepper Garlic Seasoning
- 8 Prosciutto, Sliced

Directions:
1. Preheat your Grills to 250 degrees F.
2. Pound each chicken breast with a mallet or cast iron pan so that it's about ½ inch thick.
3. On a piece of prosciutto, sprinkle mozzarella cheese and roll up. Place in the middle of a chicken breast and wrap the chicken around the prosciutto roll. Sprinkle with Lemon Pepper seasoning.
4. Smoke for an hour to 75 minutes, or until internal temperature reaches 165 degrees F.

Sweet And Sour Chicken Drumsticks

Servings: 4
Cooking Time: 150 Minutes
Ingredients:
- 3 Tbsp Brown Sugar
- 8 Chicken Drumsticks

- Garlic, Minced
- Ginger, Minced
- 2 Tbsp Honey
- 1 Cup Ketchup
- ½ Lemon Lemon, Juice
- 1/2 Lime, Juiced
- 2 Tbsp Rice Wine Vinegar
- ¼ Cup Soy Sauce
- 1 Tbsp Sweet Heat Rub

Directions:
1. In a mixing bowl, combine the ketchup, soy sauce, rice wine vinegar, brown sugar, honey, ginger, garlic, lemon, lime and Sweet Heat Rub. Reserve half of the mixture for dipping sauce and set aside. Use the remaining half and pour into a large resealable plastic bag. Add the drumsticks and seal bag. Refrigerate for a least 4-12 hours. Remove chicken from bag, discarding marinade.
2. Fire up your Pit Boss Grill and set the temperature to 225°F. If you're using a gas or charcoal grill, set it up for low-medium heat. Smoke the chicken over indirect heat with grill lid closed for 2 – 3 hours, turning once or twice, until the chicken reaches 180°F. During the last half hour, feel free to brush more glaze on.
3. Remove from grill, and let stand for 10 minutes. Feel free to add more sauce if desired or use it as a dipping sauce for the drumsticks.

Southern Fried Chicken Sliders

Servings: 8

Cooking Time: 30 Minutes

Ingredients:

- 8 Slider Buns
- ½ Cup Buttermilk
- 4 Horizontally Cut Chicken Breasts
- 2 Cups Flour, All-Purpose
- 1 Tablespoon Hot Sauce
- ¼ Cup Mayonnaise
- 2 Quarts Cooking Canola Or Soybean Oil
- ½ Cup Spicy Bread And Butter Pickle Slices
- ½ Tablespoon Champion Chicken Seasoning

Directions:

1. Fire up your Pit Boss to 350°F. If you're using a gas or charcoal grill, set it up for medium heat.
2. Place a deep cast iron pan on the grill and fill it with about 3 inches of cooking oil. Place a temperature probe into the oil.
3. While the oil heats, combine the buttermilk, hot sauce and Champion Chicken seasoning in a resealable plastic bag. Seal and shake to mix, then place the chicken in the bag and turn to coat.
4. Place the flour on a plate and dip the chicken in the flour to coat. Place the chicken on a wire rack set on a baking sheet and allow the coated chicken to set for 10 minutes, then dip again in the flour.
5. Once the oil in the cast iron pan reaches 350°F, place a temperature probe in a piece of chicken and fry the chicken, 2-3 pieces at a time. The oil temperature in the pan will drop by 25-30 degrees, so make sure not to put more than 3 pieces of chicken in the pan or your chicken will be greasy.
6. Fry the chicken until golden brown, crispy, and the internal temperature of the chicken is 170°F. Remove the chicken and place on a plate lined with paper towels.

Allow the chicken to drain and rest for 5 minutes. Fry the remaining chicken pieces, reinserting the temperature probe.

7. Once the chicken is all fried, place the chicken on the slider buns, top with spicy bread and butter pickles, and a swoop of mayo, serve immediately.

Champion Lollipop Drumsticks

Servings: 4-6

Cooking Time: 75 Minutes

Ingredients:

- 1 Cup Barbecue Sauce
- 10 Tablespoons Butter, Salted
- 12 Chicken Drumsticks
- 1 Cup Hot Sauce
- Pit Boss Champion Chicken Seasoning
- Blue Cheese Or Ranch Dressing

Directions:

1. Start up your Pit Boss. Then, set the temperature to 300°F.
2. Rinse chicken and pat dry with a paper towel.
3. Chop the very top of the drumstick on the larger, meaty side so the lollipops sit flatly. On the small end of the drumstick, about an inch above the knuckle, use a sharp knife or kitchen shears to cut the skin and tendons all the way down to the bone and pull the skin and cartilage off the knuckle.
4. Remove the tiny, sharp bone that sits right against the exposed chicken leg. Then, push all the meat and skin down to form the lollipop ball. Use your knife or shears to remove any excess tendons.
5. Season each lollipop generously with Champion Chicken seasoning and place in the aluminum pan with the flat side done and bones standing straight up. Then, cut 10 tablespoons of butter into cubes of 1 tablespoon each and place evenly throughout the rows of lollipops.

6. Cook lollipop drumsticks on your Pit Boss at 300°F for 1 hour; checking back every 20 minutes to baste the meat with the melted butter on the bottom of the pan.
7. For the Sauce: add your favorite bbq sauce into one aluminum loaf pan. Then, add 1 cup of hot sauce and 10 tablespoons of butter into the other aluminum loaf pan. Place them on the grill 5 minutes before your chicken is done. Stir well once it's warm and the butter has melted.
8. After 1 hour, use a thermometer to check the internal temperature of the lollipops. They will be ready to glaze when the temperature reaches 165°F.
9. Once ready, dip 6 lollipops in the bbq sauce and 6 in the buffalo sauce making sure to hold the leg and cover the meat entirely. Then, place the lollipops on the wing rack and put back on the grill for 15 more minutes or until the sauce is set.

Cajun Bbq Chicken

Servings: 4
Cooking Time: 25 Minutes
Ingredients:

- ½ Cup Barbecue Sauce
- ¼ Cup Beer, Any Brand
- 1 Tablespoon Butter
- 1 Pound Boneless, Skinless Chicken Breasts
- 2 Cloves Garlic Clove, Minced
- ¼ Teaspoon Ground Thyme
- 1 Teaspoon Hot Sauce
- Juice Of 1 Lime
- 1 Tablespoon Olive Oil
- ½ Teaspoon Oregano
- 2 Tablespoons Sweet Heat Rub
- 1 Tablespoon Worcestershire Sauce

Directions:

1. In a small mixing bowl, mix together the Sweet Heat Rub, oregano, and ground thyme.

2. Rub the chicken breasts all over with olive oil, making sure to completely coat the meat. Generously season the chicken breasts on all sides with the Sweet Heat mixture.
3. Fire up your Pit Boss and set the temperature to 350°F. If you're using a gas or charcoal grill, set it up for medium heat. Insert a temperature probe into the thickest part of one of the chicken breasts and place the meat on the grill. Grill the meat on one side for 10-12 minutes, then flip and grill for another 5-7 minutes, or until the chicken breasts are golden brown and juicy and reaches an internal temperature of 165°F.
4. Remove the chicken from the grill and allow to rest for 10 minutes.
5. While the chicken rests, make the sauce. Combine the butter, barbecue sauce, beer, Worcestershire sauce, lime juice, and minced garlic in a heat proof saucepan and place on the grill. Bring the sauce to a boil. Once it boils, remove it from the heat, whisk it and serve with the chicken.

Grilled Hand Pulled Chicken & White Bbq Sauce

Servings: 4
Cooking Time: 90 Minutes
Ingredients:

- 2 Tablespoons Apple Cider Vinegar
- 1 Clove Garlic, Minced
- Juice Of Half Of A Lemon
- 1 Cup Mayo
- 1 Tablespoon Olive Oil
- ½ Teaspoon Paprika, Powder
- 2 Tablespoons Sugar
- 1, 3-4 Pound Chicken, Giblets Removed And Patted Dry
- 4 Tablespoons Champion Chicken Seasoning

Directions:

1. Start up your Pit Boss. Once it's fired up, set the temperature to 350°F.
2. In a large bowl, mix all the ingredients for the sauce together. Divide the sauce between two bowls and set aside.
3. On a clean, flat surface, lay your chicken breast side down. Using the kitchen shears, remove the spine and discard. Open the chicken up and flip the chicken over so that it lays breast side up. Press the breastbone down with the heel of your hand to flatten the chicken.
4. Generously rub the chicken with the olive oil and Champion Chicken. Place on the grill, skin-side up, on the grates. Grill for 1 ½ hours, basting with half the reserved sauce every 20 minutes, until the internal temperature reaches 175°F. Remove the chicken from the grill and cover loosely for 10 minutes.
5. Shred the chicken with forks and discard the skin and bones. Serve the chicken with the remaining white BBQ sauce.

Marinated Grilled Chicken Wings

Servings: 4-6
Cooking Time: 30 Minutes
Ingredients:

- 1/2 Bottle Beer, Any Brand
- 2 Lbs Chicken Wings, Whole
- 2 Tablespoon Honey
- 1 Tablespoon Pit Boss Sweet Heat Rub
- 2 Tablespoon Rice Wine Vinegar
- 1/2 Tablesoon Sesame Oil
- 1/4 Cup Soy Sauce
- 1 Tablespoon Sriracha Hot Sauce

Directions:

1. In a large glass or plastic bowl, combine the beer, soy sauce, honey, rice wine vinegar, sriracha, sesame oil and Pit Boss Sweet Heat Seasoning. Whisk well to combine.

2. Add the chicken wings to the marinade and toss well to combine. Cover with plastic wrap and refrigerate for 2 hours and up to 24 hours.
3. Remove chicken wings from refrigerator, drain marinade and pat dry. Preheat Pit Boss Grill to 350F. Place the wings on a grill pan and grill for 20-25 minutes, or until the wings' internal temperature is 165F. Remove from the grill, serve and enjoy!

Peanut Butter And Jelly Chicken Wings

Servings: 4
Cooking Time: 35 Minutes
Ingredients:

- 1 Tsp Black Peppercorns, Ground
- 2 Tbsp Brown Sugar
- 4 Lbs Chicken Wings, Trimmed And Patted Dry
- 2 Tbsp Honey
- 1/4 Cup Peanut Butter
- 10 Oz Peanuts, Whole
- 2 Tsp Pit Boss Sweet Rib Rub
- 1/2 Red Onion, Minced
- 1/2 Cup Strawberry Preserves
- 1 Tbsp Thai Chili Sauce
- 1/4 Cup Worcestershire Sauce

Directions:

1. Place chicken wings in a 9 x13 glass baking dish. Pour mixture over chicken, cover with plastic wrap, and refrigerate for 2 hours.
2. Fire up your Pit Boss Platinum Series KC Combo and preheat grill to 400° F. Preheat griddle to medium-low flame. If using a gas or charcoal grill, set it to medium-high heat.
3. Place wings directly on grill grate, over indirect heat, and cook for 20 to 25 minutes, rotating wings every 5 minutes.

4. Meanwhile, place shelled peanuts on the griddle, turning occasionally with a metal spatula for 5 to 7 minutes, to lightly roast. Remove from the griddle and set aside to cool.
5. Remove wings from grill and allow to rest for 5 minutes. While wings are resting, shell the peanuts, and transfer to a resealable plastic bag. Use a rolling pin to crush the peanuts, then scatter peanuts on top of the chicken wings. Serve warm.

Pulled Chicken Corn Fritters

Servings: 8
Cooking Time: 45 Minutes
Ingredients:

- 2 Tsp Baking Powder
- 1 Cup Cheddar Jack Cheese, Shredded
- 1 1/2 Lbs Chicken Breast, Bone-In
- 3/4 Cup Corn Kernels, Drained
- 2 Eggs
- 3/4 Cup Flour
- 1 1/2 Tsp Lemon Juice
- 3 Tbsp Mayonnaise
- Olive Oil
- 2 Tbsp Parsley, Chopped
- 2 Tsp Pit Boss Champion Chicken Seasoning, Divided
- 1 Tbsp Scallions, Chopped
- 2 Tbsp Sour Cream
- 1 Yellow Onion, Chopped
- 1/3 Cup Milk

Directions:

1. Fire up your Platinum Series KC Combo and preheat to 425° F. If using a gas or charcoal grill, set it up for medium-high heat.
2. Remove skin from chicken breast. Drizzle chicken with olive oil, then season with 1 teaspoon of Champion Chicken. Place directly on grill grate, over indirect heat and grill for 25 minutes, until internal

temperature is 165° F. Remove from the grill and rest for 10 minutes, then pull chicken.
3. In a mixing bowl combine onion, corn, eggs, parsley, milk, cheese, and pulled chicken.
4. In a separate mixing bowl, whisk together remaining teaspoon of Champion Chicken flour and baking powder. Combine with the wet ingredients, then cover with plastic wrap and refrigerate for 2 hours.
5. Prepare dip: whisk together mayonnaise, sour cream, scallions, parsley, and lemon juice. Refrigerate until fritters are ready t serve.
6. Preheat griddle over medium-low flame.
7. Drizzle vegetable oil on the griddle, then add ¼ cup of fritter mixture to the griddl and cook 3 to 4 minutes per side, adding additional oil if needed.
8. Transfer fritters to a wire rack lined sheet tray. Allow to cool for 2 minutes, then serve warm with dip.

Cheesy Chicken

Servings: 4
Cooking Time: 45 Minutes
Ingredients:

- 4 Aged Chedder Cheese, Sliced
- 32 Oz Chicken Broth
- 1 Tsp Extra-Virgin Olive Oil
- Pit Boss Sweet Heat Rub And Grill
- 4 Plump Chicken, Boneless/Skinless

Directions:

1. Fill your hopper with your choice of pellet (we chose Competition Blend), preheat your grill to 350°F.
2. Remove the chicken from the brine. Pat the breasts dry and lightly brush olive oil on both sides of the chicken. Take your knife and slice diagonally across the top o each breast. Sprinkle a lit amount of Pit

Boss Sweet Heat Rub and Grill on each side.

3. Barbecue your chicken breasts for 30 minutes. Next, place a slice of cheddar cheese on top of each breast.

4. Heat for another 5-10 minutes or until the cheese has fully melted into the incisions you made earlier. Remove and serve for a tender chicken breast with a spicy kick and hot cheesy center. You'll receive too much credit for a recipe this easy.

Beer Can Chicken

Servings: 4
Cooking Time: 75 Minutes
Ingredients:

- 1 Beer, Can
- 1 Chicken, Whole
- Pit Boss Lemon Pepper Garlic Seasoning

Directions:

1. Preheat your Grill to 400 degrees F.
2. Season the chicken all over with spices. Open the can of your favorite pop/beer and place the opening of the chicken over the can. Make sure that the chicken can stand upright without falling over. Place on your Grill and barbecue until the internal temperature reaching 165 degrees F (about an hour).
3. Remove from grill, slice and serve hot.

Beer Brined Smoked Cornish Hens

Servings: 4
Cooking Time: 150 Minutes
Ingredients:

- 2 Tbsp Ales Pepper
- 12 Cups Beer Brine
- 2 Cornish Game Hens
- 2 Lemons

- 6 Rosemary Sprigs
- Salt & Freshly Ground Black Pepper
- 12 Thyme Sprigs

Directions:

1. Set your Pit Boss Lockhart grill to 300°F (I have found the setting the grill at 300 will keep the top smoker temp between 200°F and 215°F, this could vary depending on the air temp and general weather conditions. You want to keep the upper smoking cabinet between 200°F and 215°F) If you're using a vertical smoker, set temp to 200°F.
2. Stuff your hens with the rosemary, thyme, and lemons. Coat the skin with the ales pepper and freshly ground black pepper.
3. Truss your hens and tie a small loop at the legs so you can hang your birds. Hang them in the Lockhart smoker and insert a probe thermometer, cook to an internal temp of 155°F.
4. Remove the hens to rest. Final temp should be 160°F.
5. Serve these with some great creamed kale or charred asparagus.

Fig Glazed Chicken With Cornbread Stuffing

Servings: 10
Cooking Time: 120 Minutes

Ingredients:

- Black Pepper
- 6 Tablespoons (For The Chicken) Butter, Unsalted
- 3 Chicken, Whole
- 2 1/5 Cups (Replace With Craisins For A Different Flavor) Dried Figs, Chopped
- 1 Egg
- 2 Tablespoon Extra-Virgin Olive Oil
- 1/2 Cup Heavy Cream
- 1/2 Cup Honey
- Kosher Salt
- 4 Tablespoon Lemon, Juice
- 1/2 Onion, Chopped
- Pit Boss Champion Chicken Seasoning
- 1 1/2 Teaspoon Finely Chopped Rosemary, Fresh
- 1 Pound Sweet Italian Sausage
- 3 Cups Water, Warm

Directions:

1. Mix figs, honey, lemon juice, and warm water. Cover with plastic wrap and let figs soften for 30 minutes. Strain the figs and reserve the liquid for glaze.
2. Heat olive oil over medium heat and sauté the onions with rosemary. Add the sausage. Cook until browned. Place into a large bowl, add the cornbread and figs. Season with Pit Boss Champion Chicken Seasoning. Stir. In a separate bowl, Stir together egg, heavy whipping cream, and chicken stock. Pour over the cornbread/fig mix and stir together. Set aside.
3. Rinse chickens and pat dry. Season liberally with Pit Boss Champion Chicken Seasoning, kosher salt and black pepper. Don't forget the cavity! Stuff cavities with Stuffing. Top each Chicken with 2 tablespoons butter.
4. Preheat your Pit Boss to 300°F. Place in a roasting tray and cook until internal temp reads 165°F.
5. While chickens cook, place the fig liquid, balsamic vinegar and butter over. Reduce to thicken and baste chickens with about 160°F or 10 minutes before finished. Rest for 10 minutes. Carve and serve!

Loaded chicken Nachos

Servings: 6-8
Cooking Time: 10 Minutes

Ingredients:

- 1 Can Black Beans, Rinsed And Drained
- 1 Cup Cheddar Cheese, Shredded
- 2 Cups Chicken, Diced
- (If Desired) Cilantro
- 1 Can Corn Kernels, Drained
- (If Desired) Pickled Jalapeno Peppers
- 1/2 Tablespoon Pit Boss Champion Chicken Seasoning
- 1/2 Red Onion, Diced
- 1/2 Cup Salsa
- 1/4 Cup Sour Cream

Directions:

1. On a large sheet pan, spread out half the tortilla chips, then cover with half the shredded cheese and one cup of chicken. Sprinkle with half of Champion Chicken seasoning. Top with the rest of the tortilla chips, cheese, chicken and remaining seasoning.
2. Turn your Pit Boss Grill to 350F. Grill for 5-7 minutes, or until the cheese is melted and bubbly and everything is warmed all the way through. Remove the pan from the grill.
3. Top the nachos with the black beans, corn, diced red onion, sour cream, cilantro and pickled jalapenos. Serve and enjoy!

Grilled Honey Chipotle Chicken Wings

Servings: 4 - 8

Cooking Time: 30 Minutes

Ingredients:

- 2 Chipotles Chopped In Adobo
- 1 Apple Cider Vinegar
- 2 Tablespoons Balsamic Vinegar
- ¼ Cup Brown Sugar
- 2 ½ Lbs Chicken Wings, Trimmed And Patted Dry
- ¼ Cup Honey
- ½ Cup Ketchup
- ¼ Cup Adobo Sauce
- 2 Tablespoons Sweet Rib Rub
- 2 Teaspoons Worcestershire Sauce

Directions:

1. Fire up your Pit Boss Grill. Once it's fired up, set the temperature to 350°F. If you're using a charcoal or gas grill, set up the grill for medium high heat.
2. In a large bowl, whisk together the apple cider vinegar, ketchup, brown sugar, honey, chopped chipotle peppers with adobo sauce, balsamic vinegar, Worcestershire sauce, and Sweet Rib Rub. Whisk the glaze until it's well combined.
3. Add the wings to the glaze and place the bowl in the refrigerator. Marinade the chicken wings for up to 12 hours. Once the wings have finished marinating, remove the chicken wings from the marinade and place the chicken wings onto the wing rack.
4. Once all the wings have been placed on the wing rack, place the wing rack on the grill. Insert a temperature probe into the thickest part into one of the wings and grill the wings for 5 minutes, and then rotate the rack 180° and grill for another 5 minutes. Remove the wings once they have an internal temperature of 165°F and the juice from the chicken runs clear.
5. Remove the wings from the grill and serve immediately.

Smoked Chicken Lo Mein

Servings: 4 – 6

Cooking Time: 120 Minutes

Ingredients:

- 2 Cup Broccoli
- ¼ Cup Chicken Stock
- 6 - 8 Chicken Thighs, Boneless, Skinless
- 1 Tbsp Chili Flakes
- 1 Tsp Cornstarch
- 4, Chopped Garlic Cloves
- 3 Tbsp Hoisin Sauce, Divided
- Knob Of Fresh Ginger, Grated
- 1, Thin Red Bell Peppers, Sliced
- 1 Tbsp Rice Wine Vinegar
- 8 Scallions, Sliced
- 1 ½ Tbsp Sesame Oil, Divided
- 1 Tbsp, Toasted Sesame Seeds
- 3.5 Oz Shitake Mushrooms, Sliced Thin
- 8 Oz Snow Peas
- 3 Tbsp Soy Sauce
- 2 Tbsp Sweet Chili Sauce
- 3 Tbsp Vegetable Oil
- 1 Lb Vermicelli Noodles, Or Linguini, Cooked And Drained

Directions:

1. In a large bowl, whisk together rice wine vinegar, 1 tablespoon of Hoisin sauce, and 1 tablespoon of sesame oil. Toss chicken to coat and allow to marinate for 1 hour.
2. Fire up your Pit Boss Platinum Series KC Combo and preheat to 225° F. If using a gas or charcoal grill, set it for low, indirect heat. Place chicken directly on the grill grate and smoke for 1 ½ to 2 hours, or until the internal temperature reaches 165° F. Remove it from the smoker, cover with foil, and rest for 10 minutes, then slice thin and set aside.

3. In a glass measuring cup whisk together 2 tablespoons of Hoisin sauce, soy sauce, sweet chili sauce, chicken stock, ½ tablespoon of sesame oil, and cornstarch. Set aside.

4. Preheat griddle to medium flame, then add oil. Working quickly, sauté ginger and garlic for 15 seconds, then add bell pepper and mushrooms and continue cooking for another minute, then add in snow peas and slaw. Toss in cooked pasta, chicken, scallions, and pour sauce over. Cook for one minute until sauce thickens and is well incorporated.

5. Transfer to platter and serve hot. Sprinkle with chili flakes and sesame seeds, if desired.

Keto Chicken Crust Pizza

Servings: 4
Cooking Time: 35 Minutes
Ingredients:

- ½ Cup Alfredo Sauce
- 1 Tbsp Butter
- ¾ Lb. Shredded Chicken
- 2 Large Eggs
- 2 + 6 Divided Garlic Clove, Minced
- 1 ½ Cups Heavy Cream
- ¾ Cup Kale
- ¼ Cup Mushroom
- 1 Cup Grated Parmesan Cheese
- Pit Boss Champion Chicken Rub
- 2 Tbsp Red Onion, Diced
- ½ Tsp Salt

Directions:

1. Fire up your Pit Boss and preheat to 400° F. If using a gas or charcoal grill, set heat to medium-high heat. Place pizza stone on grill grates and allow to preheat. Line a pizza peel with parchment paper and set aside.

2. In a medium bowl, stir together the shredded chicken, grated Parmesan cheese,

minced garlic, and sea salt. Whisk the egg lightly in a small bowl then add to chicken mixture. Mix until well combined.

3. Spread the chicken crust pizza "dough" onto the parchment paper on the pizza peel, as thinly as possible (about ¼" thic

4. Using the pizza peel, transfer the parchment to the preheated pizza stone. Grill for 15 to 20 minutes, until firm and golden on the edges. Remove from the gr and let rest for 5-10 minutes.

5. Top pizza crust with alfredo sauce, kale, mushrooms, red onion and additional parmesan cheese. Return to the grill for 1 to 15 minutes, until the cheese is melted. Slice and serve!

Cajun Chicken Carbonara

Servings: 2
Cooking Time: 20 Minutes
Ingredients:

- 2 Slices Thick-Cut Bacon
- 1 Tbsp Cajun Seasoning
- 8 Oz. Chicken Breast
- 4 Egg, Yolk
- 1 Tbsp Garlic Clove, Minced
- 1 ¼ Cup Heavy Cream
- 2 Tbsp + 1 Tbsp Divided Italian Parsley
- 1 ½ Tbsp Divided Olive Oil
- ½ Cup Grated Parmesan Cheese
- ½ Tbsp Pit Boss Hickory Bacon Seasonin
- ¼ Tbsp Red Chili Flakes
- 1 Tbsp Scallions
- ½ Lb. Spaghetti

Directions:

1. Fire up your Pit Boss and preheat to 400°F. If using a gas or charcoal grill, set the temp to medium-high heat. In a medium bowl, combine chicken, Pit Boss Hickory Bacon Seasoning, Cajun seasoning, and ½ tablespoon of olive oil. Toss to combine. Set aside or place in a

bag and marinate in the refrigerator for 30 minutes to 1 hour.

2. Place tenders on preheated grill and cook for 3 minutes per side. Remove from grill and place on a cutting board to rest for 5 minutes. Slice thinly on the diagonal and set aside.

3. In a large stock pot, boil pasta per package instructions. Drain and set aside.

4. In a large skillet heat 1 tablespoon of oil over medium heat. Sauté bacon, stirring frequently, for 3 minutes or until crisp. Add garlic and cook for one minute. Lower heat to low and add in drained pasta. Using tongs, gently toss pasta to coat in oil and bacon.

5. In a mixing bowl, whisk together heavy cream, parmesan, egg yolks, and 2 tablespoons of parsley. Slowly pour over pasta, continuously stirring, as to not scramble eggs. After 2 minutes, the sauce will thicken. Add in chicken and lemon zest, and gently stir another minute. Transfer to serving dishes and garnish with additional parsley and red chili flakes.

Pulled Chicken Jalapeno Sliders

Servings: 8-10
Cooking Time: 180 Minutes
Ingredients:

- 3 Pounds Boneless Skinless Chicken Breasts
- 8-10 Slices Cheese Of Choice
- 1/2 Cup Chicken Broth
- Pickled Jalapeños
- 1 Tsp Pit Boss Smoked Infused Sweet Mesquite Jalapeno Sea Salt
- 1/2 Cup Salsa Verde
- 1 Package Slider Buns
- 3 Tablespoons Sweet Heat Rub

Directions:

1. Add the chicken breasts, chicken broth, and salsa verde to a disposable aluminum foil pan. Season everything generously with Sweet Heat and 1 tsp of Pit Boss Smoked Infused Sweet Mesquite Jalapeno Sea Salt. Cover tightly with aluminum foil.

2. Fire up your Pit Boss Grill and set the temperature to 275°F. Place the aluminum foil pan on the grill and cook for 3-4 hours, or until the chicken is completely cooked (165°F internal temperature), tender, and falling apart. Remove from the grill and let cool slightly.

3. Shred the chicken with the meat claws and toss with the Sweet Heat rub. Then, build the sliders: top the slider buns with a scoop of the pulled chicken, a slice cheese, and a few slices of pickled jalapeños. Serve immediately.

Chicken Fajita Omelet

Servings: 4
Cooking Time: 12 Minutes
Ingredients:

- 1 Cup Bell Pepper, Sliced Thin
- To Taste, Blackened Sriracha Rub Seasoning
- 2 Tbsp Butter
- 1 Cup Cheddar Jack Cheese, Shredded
- 8 Oz Chicken Breast, Boneless, Skinless, Sliced Thin
- 6 Eggs, Beaten
- 1 Tbsp Heavy Cream
- 1 Jalapeño, Minced
- 1/2 Lime
- 1 Cup Red Onion, Sliced Thinly
- 1/3 Cup Salsa Roja
- 2 Tbsp Sour Cream
- 1 Tbsp Vegetable Oil, Divided

Directions:

1. Fire up your Pit Boss Griddle and preheat to medium heat. If using a gas or charcoal grill, preheat a cast iron skillet.

2. Drizzle sliced chicken breast with 1 teaspoon oil, then season with Blackened Sriracha.

3. Drizzle the remaining oil on the griddle, then add the chicken. Sauté for 2 minutes, then add the bell peppers and onions. Season with additional Blackened Sriracha and continue to sauté another 2 minutes, then deglaze with fresh squeezed lime juice. Remove mixture from the griddle, set aside.

4. Turn the griddle down to low, then whisk the eggs (3 per omelet) and heavy cream.

5. Melt 1 tablespoon of butter on the griddle. Quickly pour the eggs over the melted butter.

6. Flip the eggs, then add ¼ cup of cheese and divide all but ½ cup of the reserved filling into the middle of each egg. Add additional cheese and some minced jalapeño. Fold the egg over to shape the omelet.

7. Transfer the omelet to a plate and top with additional filling, cheese, salsa, sour cream, and jalapeño. Serve warm.

Buffalo Chicken Pinwheels

Servings: 8
Cooking Time: 10 Minutes
Ingredients:
- 2 T Bleu Cheese, Crumbled
- ½ Cup Buffalo Wing Sauce, Divided
- 1-2, Boneless And Skinless Chicken Breast
- ½ Cup Colby Cheese, Shredded
- 4 Oz. Cream Cheese
- 4, 10" Diameter Flour Tortillas
- 2 Scallions, Thinly Sliced [Reserve 1 Tsp Of Green For Garnish]

Directions:
1. Fire up your Pit Boss Grill and preheat to 375°F. If you're using a gas or charcoal grill, set it up for medium heat. Remove chicken from refrigerator place on grill.

Grill chicken for 10 min, turning once. Allow to rest 10 minutes, then shred.

2. In a food processor, add remaining buffalo wing sauce, cream cheese, Colby cheese, bleu cheese, and scallions. Process on low for 20 seconds. Add shredded chicken breast to mixture and pulse about 8 times, or until mixture is fully combined.

3. Place tortillas on a flat work surface and divide filling into quarters. Spread mixture evenly over each tortilla with a rubber spatula.

4. Roll up tortillas and place seam side down on cutting board. Refrigerate for 10 minutes, then slice into ½ inch pieces. Transfer to serving platter and garnish with remaining scallions. Serve with extra buffalo sauce or ranch dressing.

PORK RECIPES

Healthy Hawaiian Pulled Pork

Servings: 8-10
Cooking Time: 640 Minutes
Ingredients:

- 2 Cups Aloe Leaf Juice
- 1 Tsp Coriander, Ground
- 2 Tsp Cracked Pepper
- 1 Tsp Cumin
- Dash Of Salt
- 4-6 Garlic, Cloves
- 1 (3-Inch) Ginger, Fresh
- 1-2 Limes
- 4 Cups No Sodium Added Chicken Bone Broth
- ¼ Cup Olive Oil
- 4 Tsp Paprika
- 6-8 Lbs Pork Shoulder/Butt
- 1/2 Sweet Onion
- 2 Packets Truvia To Sweeten Above Aloe Juice
- 2 Tbs Or 2 Tbs Swerve Brown Sugar Truvia – Honey Substitute

Directions:

1. Set your grill to "smoke". Once the pot catches turn the grill up to 300°F. Make sure your flame broiler is closed, you want to use indirect heat for this recipe.
2. Add all spices into a bowl (salt, paprika, cumin, coriander, pepper, onion powder if needed). Set bowl aside.
3. Grate the ginger into a separate bowl (wet ingredients bowl).
4. Mince or smash the garlic cloves into the same bowl.
5. Dice onion and add it to the ginger and garlic (if no onion sub onion powder).
6. Juice 1-2 limes and add to the "wet" ingredients bowl.
7. Add 4 cups chicken bone broth.
8. Add two cups aloe leaf juice w/lemon and add two packets Truvia to sweeten.
9. Add 1-2 tbsp Truvia honey substitute. Mix and set bowl aside.
10. Add the oil to your Pit Boss Cast Iron and coat the bottom and sides. Place the pork in the cast iron roasting pan.
11. Take your dry rub and coat the pork.
12. Pour the wet ingredients around the pork, into the Pit Boss Cast Iron Roasting Pan.
13. Cover the roasting pan with the lid and set it on your grill.
14. Check the pork every couple hours (basting if you prefer). When internal temperature reaches 195°F (after around 6 – 8 hours of cook time), it should easily start to pull apart. Don't pull apart the whole shoulder yet.
15. Remove the Pit Boss Roasting Pan from the grill and set aside to allow it to rest for 1 hour. Remove the lid to help speed cooling.
16. Once cooled, shred the pork into a separate bowl, removing the fat as you go.
17. If you want to add some of the marinade to the pork for additional flavor, make sure you skim the fat off the top first and discard.
18. Viola! Pair with fresh grilled veggies, delicious fruit or make tacos or salads! So many options for this type of protein.

Hawaiian Pulled Pork Sliders

Servings: 6 - 8
Cooking Time: 5 Minutes
Ingredients:

- ½ Cup Apple Cider Vinegar
- 1 Package Of Cabbage
- 2 Tbsp Minced Cilantro
- 1/3 Cup Green Onions, Diced
- 1 Tbsp Mango Magic
- 1 ½ Cup Mayonnaise
- 1 Cup Pineapple, Diced
- 1 Lbs Pulled Pork
- 8 Hawaiian Rolls

Directions:

1. In a large bowl mix together all of the coleslaw ingredients and let set in refrigerator for at least 2 hours.
2. Reheat the pulled pork in a microwave or grill.
3. Serve over the pulled pork on the Hawaiian rolls.

Bangers & Mash

Servings: 6 - 8
Cooking Time: 135 Minutes
Ingredients:

- Bbq Sauce
- ¼ Cup Butter
- 3 Garlic, Cloves
- 1 Onion, Chopped
- 8 Red Potatoes, Medium
- 8 Sausages, Pork
- ½ Cup Milk

Directions:

1. Using a fork, poke holes all over every red potato.
2. Cut a whole bulb of garlic in half and set aside.
3. Turn on your Pit Boss Grill and set on smoke. After the pellets ignite, set grill temp to 300°F.
4. Set the halved garlic bulb and red potatoes on the grill. Cook the garlic for 30 minutes and the potatoes for 75 minutes.
5. Turn your Pit Boss down to 250°F and allow it to settle to that temperature.
6. Peel and mash the potatoes and garlic with butter and milk until the desired smoothness is achieved.
7. Set the sausages on the grill and smoke for 1 hour.
8. Sauté sliced onions in a pan with butter and barbecue sauce to taste.
9. After 1 hour, remove the sausages and turn off the grill. Place the onions on top of the mash potatoes and the sausage on top of the onions. Add more BBQ sauce if you wish.

Pit Boss Stuffed Pork Tenderloin

Servings: 4
Cooking Time: 180 Minutes
Ingredients:

- 1 Tbsp Brown Sugar
- 1 Tbsp Chilli, Powder
- 1/8 Tbsp Cinnamon, Ground
- 3 Tbsp Honey
- 1 Tsp Paprika, Smoked
- 1 Pork, Tenderloin
- 1 Jar Salsa

Directions:

1. Start your Pit Boss Grill on Smoke with the lid open until a fire is established in the burn pot (3-7 minutes). Then set the grill to 225°F. Allow it to come to temp.
2. Arrange salsa down center of pork tenderloin. Fold in sides and roll tenderloin carefully to distribute salsa evenly.
3. Using butcher's twine or 2, 1-inch strips o aluminum foil, wrap tenderloin at both ends to secure.
4. In a bowl, combine the chili powder, brown sugar, smoked paprika, and groun cinnamon. Mix well.
5. Brush the pork tenderloin with the warmed honey. Sprinkle the rub over the entire tenderloin. When the pork is fully coated place on the grill.
6. Smoke the tenderloin for 2 ½ to 3 hours, or until the internal temperature of pork has reached 145°F internal temperature. Slice and serve immediately.

Chinese Bbq Pork Tenderloin

Servings: 4
Cooking Time: 30 Minutes
Ingredients:

- 1/4 Cup Bbq Sauce
- 2 Garlic Cloves, Minced

- 1/4 Cup Hoisin Sauce
- 2 Lbs Pork Tenderloin, Trimmed With Silver Skins Removed
- 1 Tbsp Sugar, Granulated
- 1 Tsp Sweet Rib Rub Seasoning
- 1/4 Cup Tamari
- 1/4 Cup White Wine

Directions:

1. In a glass measuring cup, whisk together the hoisin sauce, tamari, wine, garlic, sugar, and Sweet Rib Rub.
2. Place pork tenderloin in a resealable bag, then pour the marinade over the pork and allow to marinate in the refrigerator for 4 to 6 hours.
3. Fire up your Pit Boss pellet grill on SMOKE mode and let it run with lid open for 10 minutes then preheat to 400° F. If using a gas or charcoal grill, preheat to medium-high heat.
4. Remove the pork from the marinade, then pour the marinade into a grill-safe pan.
5. Place the marinade on the grill and bring to a boil for 3 minutes. Add the BBQ sauce and simmer for 2 minutes. Remove from the grill, and set aside.
6. Place the pork on the grill and cook for 18 to 20 minutes, until an internal temperature of 145° F. Flip and baste the pork with the sauce every 3 to 5 minutes.
7. Remove the pork from the grill and allow it to rest on a cutting board for 10 minutes, prior to serving warm with additional sauce.

Smoked Lasagna With Cold Smoked Mozzarella

Servings: 8-12
Cooking Time: 70 Minutes

Ingredients:

- 15 Oz. Ricotta Cheese
- 3 Cups Cold-Smoked Mozzarella, Grated Divided
- 2 Eggs
- 6 Garlic Cloves, Chopped
- 1 Tsp Garlic Powder
- 1 Cup Grated Parmesan Cheese, Divided
- 1 Lb. Italian Sausage
- 1 Tbsp Italian Seasoning
- 1 Pkg. "No-Bake" Lasagna Noodles
- 48 Oz. Marinara Sauce
- 1 Lb. Mozzarella Block
- 1 Tbsp Olive Oil
- 1 Tbsp Chopped Oregano
- ¼ Cup Italian Parsley, Chopped
- 1 Yellow Onion, Chopped

Directions:

1. In a glass bowl, mix together the eggs, Italian seasoning, garlic powder, ricotta cheese, ½ cup parmesan cheese, and 1 cup of smoked mozzarella, and 2 tablespoons of parsley. Cover and refrigerate for 1 hour.
2. Fire up your Pit Boss Lockhart Grill and preheat to 400°F. If using a gas or charcoal grill, set it up for medium-high heat. Place a cast iron skillet on the grill grates and allow to preheat.
3. Heat olive oil in skillet, then add Italian sausage and cook for 5 minutes, then add in onion and garlic, and cook an additional 3 minutes. Remove from heat and stir in 1 tablespoon of parsley and dried oregano. Set aside and reduce grill temperature to 350° F.
4. To assemble, begin by covering the bottom of a 9x13 pan with 1 cup of sauce. For the first layer, place a single layer of uncooked noodles over the sauce, followed by ⅓ of the ricotta cheese mixture, half of the Italian sausage, 1 cup of mozzarella cheese, and 1 cup of sauce. Repeat for layer two with a single layer of uncooked lasagna noodles, ⅓ of the ricotta cheese mixture, and 1 ½ cups of sauce. Repeat for layer

three with a layer of uncooked lasagna noodles, remaining ricotta mixture, remaining Italian sausage, 1 cup of sauce. For the final layer, add a layer of uncooked lasagna noodles, remaining sauce, and remaining 1 cup mozzarella plus ½ cup parmesan.

5. Transfer lasagna to grill and cook, covered with foil, for 35 minutes. Remove foil and continue cooking for 10 minutes, sprinkle with additional parmesan and parsley, if desired. Remove from grill and let stand 15 minutes before serving.

Pulled Pork Sandwich With Pretzel Bun

Servings: 4
Cooking Time: 300 Minutes
Ingredients:

- ⅓ Cup Apple Cider Vinegar
- 1 ½ Cups Bbq Sauce, Divided
- 1 Qt. Chicken Stock
- ⅓ Cup Ketchup
- 3 Tbsp Pit Boss Pulled Pork Rub, Divided
- 1, 4 Lb. Pork Shoulder, Bone In
- 4 Pretzel Buns

Directions:

1. Fire up your Pit Boss and preheat to 400°F. If using a gas or charcoal grill, set it up for medium-high heat. In a bowl, combine the apple cider vinegar, chicken stock, ketchup, and 1 tablespoon of Pit Boss Pulled Pork Rub. Whisk well to combine and set aside.
2. Season the pork shoulder with the remaining 2 tablespoons of Pulled Pork Seasoning on all sides of the pork shoulder, then place on the grill and sear on all sides until golden brown, about 10 minutes.
3. Remove the pork shoulder from the grill and place in the disposable aluminum pan. Pour the sauce over the pork shoulder. It should come about 1/3 to ½ way up the

side of the pork shoulder. Cover the top of the pan tightly with aluminum foil.

4. Reduce the temperature of your Pit Boss grill to 250°F. Place the foil pan on the grill and cook for 4 to 5 hours, or until the pork is tender and falling off the bone.
5. Remove the pork from the grill and allow to rest for 15 minutes. Drain the liquid from the pan, reserving about a cup, then shred the pork and cover with the reserved liquid. Set 3 ½ to 4 cups of pulled pork aside for sandwiches, and save the remaining for future use.
6. While pork is resting, place 1 cup of BBQ sauce in a skillet and heat to simmer. Toss in reserved shredded pork. Divide pork among 4 pretzel buns, spoon additional BBQ sauce over the top and dig in!

Bacon Wrapped Tenderloin

Servings: 5
Cooking Time: 30 Minutes
Ingredients:

- 1 Package Bacon, Thick Cut
- 1/4 Cup Maple Syrup
- 2 Tbsp Olive Oil
- 3 Tbsp Pit Boss Competition Smoked Rub
- 1 Trimmed With Silver Skin Removed Pork, Tenderloin

Directions:

1. Lay the strips of bacon out flat, with each strip slightly overlapping the other.
2. Sprinkle the pork tenderloin with 1 tablespoon of the Pit Boss Competition Smoked Rub and lay in the center.
3. Wrap with bacon over the tenderloin and tuck in the ends.
4. In a small bowl, mix the olive oil, maple syrup and remaining seasoning together and brush onto the wrapped tenderloin.
5. Preheat your Pit Boss Grill to 350°F.

6. When the grill is ready, place your tenderloin on the grill and cook, turning, for 15 minutes.

7. Increase the grill temperature to 400°F and grill for another 15 minutes or until the internal temperature is 145°F. Serve and enjoy!

moked Pork And Green Chili amales

ervings: 6-8

ooking Time: 60 Minutes

ngredients:

- 1 Boneless, Netted Pork Roast
- 1 Cup, Fresh Cilantro, Chopped
- 3 Cloves Garlic, Peeled
- 20 Dried Cornhusks
- 1 Tbsp Lime Juice
- ¼ Cup Olive Oil
- 1 Onion, Quartered
- 4 - 6 Cups Prepared Masa Harina Tamale Dough
- 3 – 4 Serrano Peppers, Deseeded
- 1 Tbsp Sweet Heat Rub
- 1 Lb. Tomatillos, Husked And Washed

irections:

1. Began by soaking the corn husks in a pan filled with water. Soak for 2 – 4 hours, or if needed, overnight.

2. Unwrap the tomatillos from their shell and place all of them into a grill basket followed by a few Serranos, deseeded, garlic cloves and 1 onion cut into quarters.

3. Fire up your Pit Boss grill and set the temperature to 400°F. If you're using a gas or charcoal grill, set it up for medium low heat, and use smoke chips to fill your grill with smoke for 15 minutes. Place the grill basket filled with your vegetables and roast them over an open flame on your Pit Boss until vegetables have become charred.

4. Place tomatillos, peppers, garlic and onions in a bowl, cover with plastic wrap, and let stand until cool enough to handle, 10 to 15 minutes.

5. Season the pork roast generously with Sweet Heat Rub and grill at 350°F for 1 hour until the roast has a nice crust on the outside.

6. While the pork roast is cooking, add a handful of cilantro, charred vegetables, 1 tbsp of Sweet Heat Rub, 1 tbsp lime juice, and ¼ cup of olive oil to a food processor. Pulse in food processor until mixture is consistent. Set aside

7. After the pork roast has been grilled for an hour, turn heat down to 275°F. Put roast in pan with about a cup of water, cover with aluminum foil and cook for another 4 hours or until the roast can be shredded. Pour chile verde sauce over shredded pork and toss to combine.

8. To being assembling tamales, place a corn husk on a work surface. Place 2-3 tablespoons of tamale dough on larger end of husk and spread into a rectangle, about ¼" thick, leaving a small border along the edge. Place large tablespoon of chili and pork filling on top of dough. Fold over sides of husk so dough surrounds filling, then fold bottom of husk up and secure closed by tying a thin strip of husk around tamale.

9. To cook tamales, place them in a large metal colander over a large stockpot filled with water. Cover and let steam for 1 hour. After the tamales have been steamed, take them off and grill them at 350°F for about 10-20 minutes until corn husks have charred marks.

Hot And Spicy Ribs

Servings: 4
Cooking Time: 300 Minutes

Ingredients:

- 2 Finely Minced Chipotle In Adobo
- 1 Cup (Any Kind) Barbecue Sauce
- 1/2 Cup Brown Sugar
- 1/4 Cup Honey
- 1/4 Cup Olive Oil
- 1 Rack St. Louis-Style Rib(S)
- 3 Tablespoons Sweet Heat Rub

Directions:

1. Remove the ribs from their packaging, drain, and pat dry. Using a paper towel, grip the membrane on the back of the ribs and pull off. Discard the membrane and paper towel.
2. In a small mixing bowl, combine the brown sugar, olive oil, honey, BBQ sauce, and chiles in adobo. Using a basting brush, brush the front and back of the ribs generously with the BBQ mixture. Save the basting brush for later along with half of the sauce.
3. Generously season the ribs with Sweet Heat rub, making sure to focus especially on the front of the ribs.
4. Fire up your Pit Boss and set the temperature to 225°F. If you're using a gas or charcoal grill, set it up for low heat. Place the ribs on the grill and smoke at 225°F for 4-6 hours making sure to baste in the sauce every 2 hours.
5. Remove from the grill and serve with additional barbecue sauce.

Bacon Wrapped Stuffed Pickles

Servings: 6
Cooking Time: 60 Minutes

Ingredients:

- 13 Strips Bacon
- 3 Bratwursts, Raw
- 1/2 Cup Colby Jack Cheese, Shredded
- 4 Oz Cream Cheese
- 13 Large Dill Pickles, Spears
- Pit Boss Hickory Bacon Rub
- 2 Scallion, Sliced Thin
- 1/4 Cup Sour Cream

Directions:

1. Fire up your Pit Boss Platinum Series KC Combo and preheat grill to 375°F.
2. Preheat griddle to medium- low flame.
3. In a mixing bowl combine cream cheese, sour cream, and scallions.
4. Use a hand mixer to blend well, then fold in grated cheddar-jack. Set aside.
5. Cook bratwurst on the griddle. Use a met spatula to chop up sausage into smaller bits and cook until browned.
6. Remove from the griddle and set aside on a sheet tray to cool.
7. Place pickles on a sheet tray. Cut in half, then remove seeds with a small measurin spoon.
8. Stuff one half of each pickle with cream cheese mixture and top with crumbled bratwurst.
9. Top with the other pickle half, then wrap in bacon.
10. Season bacon-wrapped pickles with Hickory Bacon Rub, place in cast iron skillet, then transfer to grill.
11. Grill pickles for 45 to 55 minutes, until bacon starts to crisp on top. Remove from grill. Serve warm.

Coffee-rubbed Ribs

Servings: 6 - 8
Cooking Time: 360 Minutes
Ingredients:

- 1 Tbsp Ancho Chili Powder
- Ground Black Pepper
- ½ Tsp Cocoa Powder
- 2 Tbsp Coffee
- ½ Tsp Coriander, Ground
- 1 Tbsp Dark Brown Sugar
- 1 Tsp Garlic Powder
- 2 Tbsp Kosher Salt
- 1 Tsp Onion Powder
- 1 Tsp Oregano
- 2 Tbsp Paprika
- 8 Lbs. Pork Spareribs

Directions:

1. Begin by preparing the dry rub. In a mixing bowl, whisk together the coffee, salt, paprika, brown sugar, oregano, garlic powder, onion powder, black pepper, cocoa powder and coriander. Set aside.
2. Remove the membrane from the back of your ribs: Take a butter knife and wedge it just underneath the membrane to loosen it. Using your hands or a paper towel to grip, pull the membrane up and off the bone. Place the ribs on a sheet tray, then rub each rack generously with dry rub. Wrap ribs in foil, then refrigerate overnight.
3. When ready to cook, remove ribs from the refrigerator and let come to room temp. Fire up your Pit Boss and preheat to 225°F. If using a gas or charcoal grill, set it up for low indirect heat.
4. Place foil-wrapped ribs on the grill and close lid. Cook for 4 hours then remove foil from ribs and pour accumulated juices into a glass measuring cup. Pour the sauce over the ribs, then continue to cook for an additional 1 ½ - 2 hours or until tender. Remove from grill, slice and serve.

Hawaiian Pork Butt

Servings: 8 - 10
Cooking Time: 720 Minutes
Ingredients:

- 6 - 8 Pineapple Rings
- 2 Cups Pineapple, Juice
- 1 8-10Lb Pork Butt Roast, Bone-In
- ¼ Cup Sweet Heat Rub

Directions:

1. Fire up your Pit Boss Smoker and set the temperature to 225°F. If not using a pellet smoker, set up the smoker for indirect smoking.
2. Remove the pork butt from its packaging and drain any excess liquid from the pork butt. Pat the pork butt dry with paper towels and discard the paper towels.
3. Generously season the pork butt with the Sweet Heat seasoning, making sure that the roast is coated on all sides.
4. Place the pineapple rings evenly over the pork shoulder, fat side up, and pin with toothpicks. Place the pork butt into the 9x13 pan and pour the pineapple juice over the top.
5. Set the pan into the smoker. Make sure that the pork butt is placed as close to the center of the rack as possible for even cooking.
6. Place a temperature probe into the thickest part of the pork butt, and smoke the pork until it reaches an internal temperature of 201°F. The pork should be deeply browned and smell very porky.
7. Once the pork butt reaches its internal temperature, remove the pork butt from the grill and wrap it tightly in foil. Allow the roast to rest for at least 1 hour before shredding.
8. After the roast has rested for an hour, shred the pork with your meat claws, discarding any large chunks of fat. Serve immediately.

Pork Butt With Sweet Chili Injection

Servings: 6
Cooking Time: 300 Minutes
Ingredients:

- To Taste, Blackened Sriracha Rub Seasoning
- 1/2 Tbsp Blackened Sriracha Rub Seasoning (For Injection)
- 1/4 Cup Butter, Melted
- 2 Cups Chicken Stock
- 1/2 Cup Chicken Stock (For Injection)
- 1 Tbsp Ginger Root, Sliced Thin
- 1/2 Lime, Juiced
- 1 Tbsp Olive Oil
- 5 Lbs Pork Butt, Bone-In
- 1 Red Onion, Sliced
- 1/4 Cup Rice Vinegar
- 1/2 Tbsp Sugar, Granulated
- 2 Tbsp Sweet Chili Sauce

Directions:

1. Place the pork butt on a sheet tray and pat dry with a paper towel.
2. Prepare the injection solution: Whisk together all ingredients in a glass measuring cup (1/2 cup Chicken Stock, 1/4 cup melted Butter, 1/4 cup Rice Wine Vinegar, 1/2 tbsp Blackened Sriracha Rub Seasoning, 1/2 Lime juice, 1/2 tbsp granulated Sugar).
3. Use a meat syringe to inject the solution into the pork butt, spacing every ½ inch.
4. Score the fat cap in a cross-hatch pattern, then rub sweet chili sauce on the outside of the pork butt, and season with Blackened Sriracha. Allow to sit at room temperature for 30 minutes.
5. Fire up your Pit Boss and with the lid open, set your temperature to SMOKE mode.
6. Once the fire is lit, preheat to 250° F. If using a gas or charcoal grill, set it up for low, indirect heat.
7. Place the pork shoulder on the grill grate and smoke for 2 hours.
8. Place a Dutch oven or deep cast iron skille on the grill. Heat olive oil, then add sliced onion and ginger, and set pork butt on top Pour in chicken stock, then cover with a tight lid or foil.
9. Increase temperature to 325° F, and brais for 3 hours, until pork is tender. Remove the pork from the Dutch oven, and set aside to rest on a sheet tray, or cutting board.
10. Pull pork, then serve warm with braising jus.

Dry Rub Smoked Ribs

Servings: 4
Cooking Time: 300 Minutes
Ingredients:

- 1 Rack Baby Back Rib
- 1 Tablespoon Olive Oil
- Pit Boss Sweet Heat Rub

Directions:

1. Start your Pit Boss on "smoke". Once it's fired up, set the temperature to 225°F.
2. Remove the membrane from the back of the ribs. Rub the ribs down with olive oil, then generously coat both sides with Swee Heat Rub. For deeper flavor penetration, gently pat the spices into the meat and let sit in the refrigerator for at least an hour.
3. Smoke the ribs for about 5 hours or until the temperature is between 180°F and 195°F, and the meat is dark, glossy and easily tears apart.
4. When the ribs are finished, remove from the grill and let them rest for 5 minutes before serving.

Raspberry Spiral Ham

Servings: 12

Cooking Time: 120 Minutes

Ingredients:

- 1 Ham, Spiral (Precooked)
- Pit Boss Raspberry Chipotle Spice Rub
- 1/2 Jar Raspberry Jam
- 1 Quart Raspberry, Fresh
- 1/4 Cup Sugar
- 1/3 Cup Water, Warm

Directions:

1. Preheat your Grill to 225F.
2. Season the ham with Raspberry Chipotle Spice, taking care to season in between each slice. Place in your Grill and smoke for about 2 hours.
3. Just before you pull the ham, combine glaze ingredients in a saucepan over medium heat until raspberries are no longer whole and the glaze is runny. If you want a smoother glaze, remove the raspberry seeds by draining the glaze through cheesecloth.
4. Pour glaze over the ham just before serving. Slice and serve hot. Enjoy!

Cheesy Potato Stuffed Pork Chops

Servings: 4

Cooking Time: 45 Minutes

Ingredients:

- 4 Bone-In Pork Chops
- 1 Package Frozen Shredded Hash Browns, Thawed
- 1 Tbsp Parsley, Minced Fresh
- Pulled Pork Seasoning
- 1 Cup Shredded Cheddar Cheese
- ¼ Cup Sour Cream
- White Onion, Diced

Directions:

1. Place the pork chops on a flat work surface. Using a sharp knife, cut a pocket into the side of each pork chop, being careful not to cut all the way through the sides of the chop. Season the pork chops generously on both sides with Pulled Pork Seasoning.
2. In a large mixing bowl, mix together the hash browns, shredded cheddar, sour cream, diced onion, parsley, and 1 tablespoon of Pulled Pork seasoning. Stuff each pork chop with about ¼ cup of the potato filling. Use a toothpick to securely close the chop if needed.
3. Fire up your Pit Boss and set the temperature to 350°F. If you're using a gas or charcoal grill, set it up for medium heat. Insert a temperature probe into the thickest part of one of the chops and place the meat on the grill. Grill the chops on one side for 10-15 minutes, then flip and grill for another 10-15, or until the internal temperature of the chops reach 145°F.
4. Remove the chops from the grill, take the toothpicks out of the meat, and serve immediately.

Bbq Pork Chops With Bourbon Glaze

Servings: 4

Cooking Time: 30 Minutes

Ingredients:

- 4 8-To-10-Ounce Bone-In Pork Loin Chops, Trimmed Of Excess Fat
- 1/2 Cup Brown Sugar
- 2 Garlic Clove, Minced
- 2 Tbsp Honey
- 1 Cup Ketchup
- 1/4 Cup Molasses
- Sweet Rib Rub Seasoning
- 2 Tbsp Worcestershire Sauce

Directions:

1. First, place pork chops onto sheet pan lined with butcher paper. Season generously with Sweet Rib Rub, making

sure to coat all sides of the chops. Set aside while you make the glaze.

2. In a medium sized mixing bowl, combine the ketchup, brown sugar, molasses, honey, garlic, Worcestershire, and 1 tbsp Sweet Rib Rub. Mix well, add 1 shot of bourbon, mix again until sauce becomes smooth. Transfer sauce into an oven proof sauce pan.

3. Fire up your Pit Boss Grill and set the temperature to 375°F. If you're using a gas or charcoal grill, set it up for medium direct heat.

4. Grill the pork chops for 10-15 minutes per side. Place the saucepan on the grill and allow the sauce to come to a boil. Glaze the chops on both sides and let the glaze caramelize onto the chops.

5. Grill the pork chops until they are lightly charred and reach an internal temperature of 145°F - 165°F. Remove the pork chops from the grill and allow them to rest for 5 minutes.

6. Once the pork chops have finished resting, glaze them again if you choose to. Serve immediately.

Basic Smoked Ribs

Servings: 4
Cooking Time: 315 Minutes
Ingredients:
- 2 Racks Baby Back Rib
- Pit Boss Sweet Rib Rub

Directions:
1. Preheat your Pit Boss Pellet Grill to 225°F.
2. Remove the membrane on the reverse side of the ribs by sliding a butter knife under the membrane and breaking it. With a piece of paper towel, grab the broken membrane and peel back until the entire membrane is removed.
3. Season both sides of the ribs with Sweet Rib Rub.

4. Place the ribs, meat side up, on the grates of the grill and close the lid. Smoke for about 4 1/2 hours.
5. Wrap in foil and return to the grill at 350°F for another 45 minutes.
6. Pull your ribs off the grill and rest for 10 minutes.
7. Slice and serve hot. Enjoy!

Breaded Pork Chops

Servings: 6
Cooking Time: 10 Minutes
Ingredients:
- 2 Tbsp Apple Cider Vinegar
- 1 Tbsp Brown Sugar
- 2 Tbsp Butter
- 1/8 Tsp Cayenne Pepper
- 2 Eggs, Beaten
- 1/2 Cup Flour
- 1/2 Tbsp Horseradish
- 1/2 Lemon, Juiced
- 1/2 Cup Mayonnaise
- 1 1/2 Cup Panko Breadcrumbs
- 6 Pork Chops, Bone-In
- 1 Tbsp Smoked Hickory Sea Salt
- 1/4 Cup Sour Cream
- 1/2 Tbsp Stone Ground Mustard
- 1/2 Cup Vegetable Oil

Directions:
1. Place pork chops on a sheet tray, blot dry with a paper towel, then season with Smoked Hickory & Honey Sea Salt.
2. Place flour, beaten egg and bread crumbs in 3 separate bowls. Dip each pork chop in flour, then beaten egg, then breadcrumbs then set aside.
3. Prepare the Alabama White Sauce: In a small bowl, whisk together the mayonnaise, sour cream, apple cider vinegar, brown sugar, spicy brown mustard, horseradish, lemon juice, and

cayenne. Whisk until fully combined, then set aside.

4. Fire up your Pit Boss Griddle and set it to medium heat. then add the oil. When oil begins to smoke, add the butter to melt, then lay out the pork chops. Cook pork chops 2 to 3 minutes per side until golden brown and crisp. For thicker chops, add 1 minute per side.

5. Serve breaded pork chops warm with Alabama White Sauce.

Next Level Smoked Porchetta

Servings: 6

Cooking Time: 360 Minutes

Ingredients:

- 1 Tbs Ancho Chili Powder
- 1/2 Cup Brown Sugar
- 3 Tbs Grilling Seasoning
- 1 Tbs Chopped Italian Parsley
- 1/2 Cup Maple Syrup
- 1 Tsp Dry Oregano
- 1 Tbs Chopped Oregano, Leaves
- 1/2 Pork, Belly (Skinless)
- 1 Whole Pork, Tenderloins
- 6 Slices Prosciutto, Sliced
- 1 Tbs Chopped Rosemary, Fresh
- 1 Tbs Chopped Sage, Leaves
- 1/2 Cup Sugar, Cure

Directions:

1. Sprinkle Sugar Cure on each side and rub in. (You can cure pork belly without using Sodium Nitrite (in the cure mix) but it is much safer if you use it, so I definitely recommend it).

2. In a small bowl, mix brown sugar, maple syrup, ancho chili powder and oregano, and whisk. Slather on both sides of each pork belly piece.

3. Place pork bag (if you can find a 2 gallon or larger one) or container and refrigerate Rotate and flip each 24 hours.

4. After 3 days remove pork belly and rinse each piece thoroughly.

5. If you do not rinse well the porchetta (or bacon) will be too salty due to the sugar cure.

6. Lay pork belly skin side down on a large cutting board.

7. Lightly score the meat side with diamond cuts to allow the seasoning to penetrate.

8. Lightly sprinkle with grilling seasoning, then coat well with the herb mix.

9. Lay out the prosciutto, then lay the pork tenderloin on the pork belly.

10. Lightly sprinkle tenderloin with seasoning, and wrap the pork belly tightly around it.

11. Use cooking twine to tie up tightly.

12. Season the exterior of the pork belly lightly but evenly with grilling seasoning.

13. Place in smoker with apple wood pellets (recommended) at 250°F.

14. Smoke for 6 hours, or until internal temperature reaches around 175°F.

15. Remove and allow to rest for 20 minutes. Once it cools, then slice thinly and sear in a hot skillet.

16. Let it cool again for about 10 minutes before serving.

Grilled Pork Tenderloin

Servings: 4
Cooking Time: 20 Minutes

Ingredients:

- 2 Tablespoons Brown Sugar
- 2 Tablespoons Olive Oil
- 2 Tablespoons Pit Boss Tennessee Apple Butter Seasoning
- 1 Pork Tenderloin, Trimmed With Silver Skins Removed

Directions:

1. In a small bowl, combine the olive oil, brown sugar, and Tennessee Apple Butter seasoning until well combined. Generously rub the pork tenderloin with the mixture. Allow the pork tenderloin to marinade for 1 hour.
2. Start your Pit Boss on smoke. Once it's fired up, set the temperature to 350°F.
3. Grill the tenderloin for 5-7 minutes on each side, flipping the tenderloin only once and cooking until the internal temperature reaches 140-145°F.
4. Remove the tenderloin from the grill and allow to rest 10 minutes before slicing and serving.

Pork Belly Chili Con Carne

Servings: 4
Cooking Time: 120 Minutes

Ingredients:

- Avocado, Diced
- 2 Bay Leaves
- 1 Lbs Beef Stew Meat
- 12 Oz Beef Stock
- 12 Oz Beer, Bottle
- 15 Oz Black Beans, Rinsed And Drained
- 3 Tbsp Chili Powder
- Cilantro, Chopped
- 1 Tsp Coriander, Ground
- 2 Tsp Cumin, Ground
- 1 Tbsp Flour
- 4 Garlic Cloves, Minced
- 2 Tsp Mexican Oregano, Dried
- 2 Tbsp Olive Oil
- 2 Oz Pancetta, Diced
- Pork Belly, Cut Into 1 Inch Chunks
- 2 Red Onion, Chopped
- Rice, Cooked
- To Taste, Salt & Pepper
- Scallion, Sliced Thin
- 1/4 Cup Tomato Purée

Directions:

1. Fire up your Pit Boss pellet grill on SMOKE mode and let it run with lid open for 10 minutes then preheat to 425°F. If using a gas or charcoal grill, set it up for medium-high heat. Place Dutch oven on grill and allow to preheat.
2. Heat the olive oil in the Dutch oven, then sauté the pancetta until crisp. Add the onions and sauté for 3 minutes, then add the garlic and sauté 1 minute, until fragrant. Remove mixture with a slotted spoon and set aside.
3. Add the pork belly and beef to the pot to brown, then add the chili powder, cumin, oregano, and coriander. Add the flour and cook for 2 minutes, stirring constantly.
4. Add the beer, beef stock, and tomato purée. Stir well, then return the pancetta mixture to the pot. Add the black beans and bay leaves, then season with salt and pepper.
5. Bring chili to a simmer, then reduce temperature to 325°F and simmer, uncovered, for 2 hours, stirring occasionally, until meat is tender, and sauce has thickened.
6. Remove the chili from the grill, then serve warm with cooked rice, avocado, fresh cilantro, and scallions.

Beer Braised Pork Belly

Servings: 4

Cooking Time: 90 Minutes

Ingredients:

- 1, Dark Beer, Any Brand
- 3 Cups Broth, Beef
- 1 Tablespoon Chinese Cooking Wine (Such As Shaoxing) Or Dry Sherry Wine
- 1 Teaspoon Chinese Five Spice Powder
- 2, Smashed Garlic, Cloves
- 1 Inch Knob Ginger, Peeled And Thinly Sliced
- 1 Onion, Sliced
- 2 Pounds Pork Belly, Cut Into 1 Inch Chunks
- 2 Tablespoons Rice Wine Vinegar
- 2 Tablespoons, Dark Soy Sauce, Low Sodium
- 3 Tablespoons Sugar

Directions:

1. Place a heavy dutch oven on a stovetop over medium high heat. Add the pork belly and brown on all sides, about 5 minutes. Once the pork belly has browned, add in the onion, ginger, and garlic, and stir well.
2. Pour the beer, beef broth, soy sauce, dark soy sauce, sugar, Chinese cooking wine, rice wine vinegar, and Chinese five spice powder into the pan. Place a lid on the pan and bring it to a boil. Once it boils, remove it from the heat.
3. Fire up your Pit Boss Grill and set the temperature to 325°F. Place the pan of pork belly on the grill and braise for 1 ½ hours, or until the pork belly is falling apart tender and glazed.
4. Remove the pork belly from the grill and serve immediately.

3-2-1 St. Louis Ribs

Servings: 4

Cooking Time: 360 Minutes

Ingredients:

- 1/2 Cup Brown Sugar
- 6 Tbsp Butter
- 1 Cup Memphis Style Bbq Sauce
- To Taste, Pulled Pork Rub
- 2 St. Louis Style Rib Racks

Directions:

1. Fire up your Pit Boss and with the lid open, set your temperature to SMOKE mode.
2. Once the fire is lit, preheat to 200° F. If using a gas or charcoal grill, set it up for low, indirect heat.
3. Remove the membrane on the back of the ribs, trim off excess fat, meat flap, and silverskin, then season both sides of the ribs with Pulled Pork Rub. Transfer to the grill and smoke for 3 hours.
4. Remove ribs from the grill, and set on 2 sheets of Pit Boss Butcher paper. Sprinkle with the brown sugar, top with the butter cut into small pads, and then wrap the ribs.
5. Return the ribs to the grill and increase temperature to 225° F. Cook for 2 hours.
6. Remove the ribs from the grill and carefully cut open the paper with scissors, being cautious of hot steam.
7. Fold over the paper, baste with Memphis-style sauce, then return ribs to the grill (meat side up). Close the lid and cook ribs another hour, until tender.
8. Remove ribs from the grill, allow to rest for 15 minutes, then slice and serve hot.

Egg & Bacon French Toast Panini

Servings: 2
Cooking Time: 10 Minutes
Ingredients:

- 6 Bacon Slices
- 1 Tbsp Black Pepper
- 4 Brioche Sandwich Slices, Day Old
- 2 Tbsp Butter
- 1 Tbsp Cinnamon-Sugar
- 6 Eggs
- 1 Tbsp Heavy Cream
- 1 Tbsp Maple Syrup
- 1 Tbsp Salt

Directions:

1. Fire up your Pit Boss KC Combo Grill and preheat griddle to 375°F. If using a gas or charcoal grill, set heat to medium heat. For all other grills, preheat cast iron skillet on grill grates.
2. Place butter on griddle and spread to coat surface.
3. In a pie plate, whisk together 2 eggs, heavy cream, and maple syrup.
4. Soak both sides of bread slices in egg mixture and transfer to griddle. Cook for 2 minutes, flipping halfway until egg mixture is cooked and golden. Set aside.
5. Lay bacon on the griddle, and cook 3 minutes per side, until golden.
6. Transfer to lower right-hand corner of griddle to keep warm.
7. Crack 4 eggs on top of rendered bacon fat. Season with salt and pepper. Cook 1 minute per side, or to desired doneness.
8. Lay eggs on top of French toast, add bacon, then place the other slice of French Toast on top.
9. Transfer back to griddle for another minute to warm, sprinkle with extra cinnamon-sugar, then slice in half and serve hot.

Apple Cider & Maple Glazed Ham

Servings: 10 - 14
Cooking Time: 190 Minutes
Ingredients:

- 1 1/2 Cups Apple Cider
- 3 Tbsp Apple Cider Vinegar
- 1/2 Cup Packed Light Brown Sugar
- 2 Tbsp Unsalted Butter
- ¼ Tsp Chili Powder
- 2 Tsp Cornstarch
- 3 Tbsp Dijon Mustard
- ½ Tsp Ground Cinnamon
- ¼ Tsp Ground Cloves
- Large Cast Iron Skillet
- 1/2 Cup Pure Maple Syrup
- 2 Tsp Pit Boss Tennessee Apple Butter Rub
- 1 Spiral-Sliced Ham, Bone-In
- ¼ Tsp Thyme, Dried
- 3 Tbsp Yellow Mustard

Directions:

1. Remove ham from refrigerator and let rest at room temperature for 2-3 hours.
2. Fire up your Pit Boss grill and preheat to 300° F. If using a gas or charcoal grill, set heat to medium-high heat.
3. Create a bed of foil in the bottom of a large cast iron pan, making sure to have enough to seal entire ham. Set ham inside foil and add one cup of water to the bottom of pan. Pour some glaze (about ⅓ of mixture) over ham, making sure to coat in between slices. Wrap ham tightly in foil and grill for 2 hours.
4. Remove ham from grill and increase temperature to 400° F. Carefully unfold foil to expose ham and pour an additional ⅓ of glaze over ham. Leave ham exposed and grill for 30 minutes or until edges are golden brown and caramelized.
5. Remove ham from grill and carefully remove foil from underneath ham, so that

ham is directly sitting on cast iron. Return to grill, brush with more glaze, and grill another 15 minutes. Remove ham from grill, let rest for 15 minutes, then carve and serve with remaining glaze.

Smoked St. Louis Style Ribs With Tequila Bbq

Servings: 8
Cooking Time: 240 Minutes
Ingredients:

- 1/2 Cup Brown Sugar
- 2 Garlic, Cloves
- 3 Tbsp Honey
- 1 Cup Ketchup
- 1/2 Squeezed Lime
- 3 Tbsp Molasses
- 1 Jar Mustard
- 2 Slabs Slabs St. Louis-Style Rib Racks
- 1 Bottle Sweet Heat Rub
- 1/4 Cup Tequila Blanco

Directions:

1. First, make the barbecue sauce. In a mixing bowl, add the ketchup, brown sugar, garlic cloves, molasses, honey, tequila, lime, and 1 tbsp Sweet Heat Rub. Mix together well until glaze is blended together. Set aside.
2. Prepare the ribs. Pat the ribs dry with paper towels, then pull the thin membrane off the back of the ribs and discard. Using a basting brush, coat the meat on both sides with a thin layer of mustard and season heavily with Sweet Heat Rub until the ribs are completely coated. Repeat with the second rack of ribs. Place the ribs on a baking sheet and refrigerate overnight, or for 12 hours if you choose to.
3. Once the ribs have finished marinating, remove them from the refrigerator and set out two sheets of large, heavy duty aluminum foil. Place one rack of ribs on

each sheet of foil, meat-side down, and fold the edges over to form a sealed pouch.
4. Fire up your Pit Boss Grill and set the temperature to 225°F. If you're using a gas or charcoal grill, set it up for low, indirect heat. Place the rib packets on the grill, meat-side up, and smoke for 2-3 hours, or until the ribs are nearly tender.
5. Remove the ribs from the grill and take the aluminum foil off the ribs and place them back onto the grill for another hour. Brush generously with the tequila barbecue sauce on both sides, then grill for 5 minutes, meat- side up. Baste the ribs one more time with the barbecue sauce, then flip them meat-side down and grill for a final 5 minutes. The ribs should be sticky and caramelized. Remove the ribs from the grill and serve immediately with the remaining barbecue sauce.

Kansas City Style Championship Ribs

Servings: 4
Cooking Time: 210 Minutes
Ingredients:

- Apple Juice
- 2 Racks Baby Back Rib
- 2 Cups Brown Sugar
- 24 Oz Dijon Mustard
- 4 Tbsp Pit Boss Sweet Rib Rub
- Spray Bottle

Directions:

1. Pour Dijon Mustard into a mixing bowl. Mix in brown sugar until mustard taste diminishes and a sweet taste takes over.
2. Generally, you will use a half bag of brown sugar for 2 bottles and the whole bag for 4 bottles. The key is for the tangy mustard taste to turn sweet.
3. When this mix is brushed on the ribs the mix of pork flavor and this glaze will produce a sweet and sassy result. The

easiest way to mix is with an electric mixer but a whisk will do nicely. This will become very thick and sticky.

4. Pre-heat Grill for 10 minutes and then set cooking temperature to 275°.

5. Place ribs, back side down, on the cooking grid. Note: If you are doing multiple slabs, I suggest you use a rib rack. Most Rib Racks will hold 6 slabs. This will allow ribs to cook evenly. The rib rack allows for more slabs since ribs will sit in rack on their edge. Try to put meatier side up.

6. Spray ribs thoroughly with apple juice every 30-40 minutes. Apple Juice not only helps to keep meat moist and juicy while cooking, the acidity also helps to break down the muscles, thus tenderizing as well. I have had people tell me they prefer Pineapple juice or a mixture of apple and pineapple. Personally, I can't tell the difference, but you can experiment for yourself if you want to. The result will be same.

7. Note: How to tell when ribs are done? It is hard to measure temp of a rib with a meat thermometer due to the meat between the bones being so tight. You can get a false reading if the thermometer is touching a bone. Take your tongs and pick up slab in the middle. If the rib folds over and is limp and the meat just begins to pull away from the bone, they are done.

8. Remove ribs from grill and place in a pan (long enough for ribs to fit)

9. Glaze both sides of ribs with a light coat of the sassy glaze. This is a flavor enhancer, not a cover up. Just a light coat is plenty. If you really like the glaze there will generally always be some left over, and you can add to your desire while on the plate.

10. Wrap ribs in foil and let stand for 15 minutes

11. Serve (you can serve in slab form and let each guest cut his own or I like to cut ribs and serve as single bones.

12. Enjoy!

Raspberry Chipotle Pork Kebabs

Servings: 8
Cooking Time: 15 Minutes
Ingredients:

- 1/8 Cup Vinegar Apple Cider
- 3 Green Bell Pepper, Sliced
- 1 Tbsp Honey
- 1 Tbsp Olive Oil
- 2 Tbsp Pit Boss Raspberry Chipotle Spice Rub
- 1 Lb Pork, Loin (Boneless)
- 1 Red Onion, Chunked
- 8 (12 Inch) Skewers

Directions:

1. In a medium bowl, whisk together apple cider vinegar, Raspberry Chipotle seasoning, olive oil, and honey. Add the cubed pork loin to marinade and toss to coast. Cover with plastic wrap and let marinate for 30 minutes to 1 hour.

2. Once meat is marinated, remove from marinade and thread cubed pork loin onto the skewers, alternating with pieces of bell pepper and red onion.

3. Light ceramic charcoal barbecue to 400*F. Grill kebabs directly on the grill, turning often, until all sides of the meat is well browned and vegetables are tender (about 15 minutes).

4. Serve immediately. Note: If using wood skewers, soak in water for 30-45 minutes prior to use.

Apple Bacon Smoked Ham With Glazed Carrots

Servings: 8-12
Cooking Time: 120 Minutes
Ingredients:

- 1 1/2 Cup Apple Cider
- 3 Tablespoon Apple Cider Vinegar
- 2 Apples
- 1 Lb. Bacon
- 2 Tablespoon Butter, Unsalted
- 2 Tablespoon Cornstarch
- 3 Tablespoon Dijon Mustard
- Pit Boss Smoke Infused Applewood Bacon Rub
- 1/2 Cup Pure Maple Syrup
- 1 Large Bone In Spiral Cut Smoked Ham
- 2 Tablespoon Yellow Mustard

Directions:

1. Turn your grill to smoke mode, let the fire catch and then set to 250 degrees F (121 degrees C).
2. Smoke the bacon directly on the grates for 25 minutes, flipping at the 15-minute mark. Thinly slice the apples while the bacon cooks. Once the bacon is done, set your temperature down to 225 degrees F (107 degrees C).
3. Put the spiral-sliced ham into an aluminum foil roasting pan. Start by adding apple into the first slice and every other slice after that. Fill in all other slices with the bacon strips. Season with Pit Boss Smoke Infused Applewood Bacon Rub. Add any extra apple cider to the bottom of the pan for added flavor.
4. Place ham in the grill for 60 minutes.
5. Meanwhile, in a saucepan, whisk together apple cider, maple syrup, apple cider vinegar, Dijon mustard, yellow mustard, cornstarch and Pit Boss Smoke Infused Applewood Bacon Rub. Bring to a boil. Reduce to a simmer, stirring often, until the sauce has thickened and reduced (approximately 15-20 minutes). Stir in the butter until it has completely melted. Glaze should thicken more as it stands.
6. After 60 minutes, add carrots into the roasting pan and glaze the entire ham. Glaze again every 30 minutes until done.
7. Remove ham from grill and allow to rest covered with foil for 20 minutes before serving.
8. Serve with remaining warmed up sauce if desired.

Smoked Homemade Breakfast Sausage Links

Servings: 3-6
Cooking Time: 90 Minutes
Ingredients:

- ½ Tsp Black Pepper
- 1 Tbsp Brown Sugar
- Ice Water Dried Marjoram
- ⅛ Tsp Ground Cloves
- ⅓ Cup Ice Water
- 20/22 Mm Natural Sheep Casings
- Pit Boss Tennessee Apple Butter Rub
- 2Lbs. Pork Sausage, Ground

Directions:

1. One hour before stuffing, rinse sheep casings thoroughly and let soak in warm water for 60 minutes.
2. In a chilled stand mixing bowl, add the pork sausage, Tennessee Apple Butter, marjoram, cloves, brown sugar, and ice water. Use the paddle attachment and mix on low speed for 5 minutes, until threads appear in the meat. Place mixture in the refrigerator while preparing the sausage stuffer.
3. Thread the sausage stuffer with the prepared sheep casings, then fill the well with the meat mixture. Use one hand to hold the wand to press the meat through the auger, and the other hand guide and fill the casings being careful to avoid air

gaps while also not overstuffing the casings.

4. Twist the sausages into 4 to 5-inch links, twisting every other link. Use a sausage pricker to prick any air bubbles out of the links.

5. Place sausage links on a sheet tray and refrigerate overnight.

6. Fire up your Pit Boss Lockhart Grill and set it to Smoke mode. If using a gas or charcoal grill, set it up for low indirect heat.

7. Hang sausage links on S-hooks and place in the smoking cabinet. Increase temperature to 350°F. Smoke links for 1 hour, then increase the temperature to 425°F and cook for another 30 minutes.

8. Remove links from the cabinet and serve hot. For additional browning, sear in cast iron, 1 minute per side.

Grilled Tacos Al Pastor

Servings: 8
Cooking Time: 15 Minutes
Ingredients:

- 2 Tsp Annatto Powder
- Cilantro, Chopped
- Corn Tortillas
- 2 Tsp Cumin
- 1 Tsp Granulated Garlic
- 2 Tbsp Guajillo Chili Powder
- Jalapeno Pepper, Minced
- Lime, Wedges
- 1 Tsp Oregano, Dried
- 1/2 Tsp Pepper
- 1/2 Cup Pineapple, Juice
- 1/2 Pineapple, Skinned & Cored
- 2 Lbs Pork Shoulder, Boneless, Sliced Thin
- 1 1/2 Tsp Salt
- 2 Tbsp Tomato Paste
- 2 Tbsp Vegetable Oil
- 1/4 Cup White Vinegar

- Yellow Onion, Chopped

Directions:

1. Prepare marinade: In a mixing bowl, whisk together pineapple juice, vinegar, tomato paste, chili powder, annatto, cumin, granulated garlic, oregano, salt, and pepper. Set aside.

2. Slice pork shoulder into thin slices (around ¼" thick), then place in a resealable plastic bag. Pour marinade over pork, seal bag, and turn to coat. Refrigerate overnight.

3. Fire up your Pit Boss grill and preheat to 450° F. If using a gas or charcoal grill, set it up for high heat.

4. Remove the pork from the marinade and set on the grill. Grill over high heat for 3 5 minutes, turning frequently. Transfer to a cutting board to rest for 10 minutes, the slice thin.

5. Grill pineapple for 3 minutes, turning one Set aside on a cutting board, and chop once cooled.

6. Assemble tacos: tortillas, pork, pineapple jalapeño, onion, and cilantro. Serve warm with fresh lime wedges.

Bbq Smoked Pork Loin

Servings: 4

Cooking Time: 120 Minutes

Ingredients:

- 1 Tbsp Olive Oil
- Pit Boss Pulled Pork Rub
- 3 Lbs Pork Loin, Center-Cut

Directions:

1. Fire up your Pit Boss pellet grill and preheat to 250°F. If using a gas or charcoal grill, set it up for low, indirect heat.
2. Score the fat cap of the loin in a cross-hatch pattern, then drizzle with olive oil, and season with Pit Boss Pulled Pork Rub.
3. Transfer the pork directly on the grates. Smoke for 1 ½ to 2 hours, until the internal temperature reaches 145°F.
4. Remove the pork loin from the gill and rest for 15 minutes, before slicing and serving warm.

Bacon Wrapped Asparagus

Servings: 4

Cooking Time: 30 Minutes

Ingredients:

- 1 Bunch Asparagus
- 1 Package Bacon

Directions:

1. Set grill to 400°F.
2. Lay one piece of bacon on a clean surface.
3. Starting from the bottom, roll the bacon around one piece of asparagus. Repeat for all pieces of bacon.
4. Place bacon wrapped asparagus on your grill for about 25 minutes, or until the bacon is cooked. Rotate the asparagus so that the bacon cooks evenly. Serve hot.

Pulled Pork

Servings: 6 - 8

Cooking Time: 300 Minutes

Ingredients:

- 1/3 Cup Apple Cider Vinegar
- 4 Cups Chicken Broth
- 1/3 Cup Ketchup
- 2 Tbsp Pit Boss Pulled Pork Seasoning
- 4 Lbs. Pork Shoulder, Bone In

Directions:

1. Preheat your Pit Boss grill to 350°F. In a bowl, combine the chicken broth, ketchup, apple cider vinegar, and 1 tablespoon of Pulled Pork Seasoning. Whisk well to combine and set aside.
2. Generously season the pork shoulder with the remaining 3 tablespoons of Pulled Pork Seasoning on all sides of the pork shoulder, then place on the grill and sear on all sides until golden brown, about 10 minutes.
3. Remove the pork shoulder from the grill and place in the disposable aluminum pan. Pour the chicken broth mixture over the pork shoulder. It should come about 1/3 to ½ way up the side of the pork shoulder. Cover the top of the pan tightly with aluminum foil.
4. Reduce the temperature of your Pit Boss grill to 250°F. Place the foil pan on the grill and grill for four to five hours, or until the pork is tender and falling off the bone.
5. Remove the pork from the grill and allow to cool slightly. Drain the liquid from the pan, reserving about a cup, then shred the pork and cover with the reserved liquid. Serve and enjoy!

BAKING RECIPES

Chocolate Bacon Cupcakes

Servings: 12
Cooking Time: 120 Minutes
Ingredients:

- 1 Lb Bacon
- 1 1/2 Tsp Baking Powder
- 1 1/2 Tsp Baking Soda
- 1 Cup Cocoa, Powder
- 2 Egg
- 1 3/4 Cups Flour
- 1 Cup Milk, Whole
- 1/2 Cup Oil
- 1 Tsp Salt
- 2 Cups Sugar
- 2 Tsp Vanilla

Directions:

1. Start your Pit Boss on SMOKE with the lid open until a fire is established in the burn pot (3-7 minutes). Preheat to 250°F.
2. Once your grill is preheated, place bacon strips on the grates. Smoke for 1hr-1 ½ hours or until desired crispiness is achieved.
3. Remove the bacon from the grill and set aside.
4. Increase set the temperature to 350°F and preheat.
5. Mix the rest of the ingredients in a bowl with an electric mixer until it is nice and smooth.
6. Pour the mixture into a cupcake tin.
7. Transfer the tin to your grill and bake for about 20 - 25 minutes.
8. Allow the cupcakes to cool on a wire rack. Once cooled, top with your favorite premade icing and a half of strip of the bacon. Serve and enjoy!

Sweet And Spicy Baked Beans

Servings: 20
Cooking Time: 120 Minutes
Ingredients:

- 1 - 21 Oz Apple Pie Filling, Can
- 1 Gallon Baked Beans
- 1 Tbs Chilli, Powder
- 1 Green Bell Pepper, Diced
- 1 10 Oz Drained Jalapeno, Can Diced
- 1 Cup Maple Syrup
- 1 Onion, Diced
- 1 Lb Pork, Pulled

Directions:

1. Start Grill at 350 degrees.
2. Place all ingredients in mixing bowl and mix well.
3. Pour bean mixture into foil pans.
4. Bake in grill till bubbling throughout – about 2 hours.
5. Rest at least 15 minutes before serving.

Chocolate Peanut Butter Cookies

Servings: 4
Cooking Time: 12 Minutes
Ingredients:

- 1/2 Tsp Baking Soda
- 1/2 Cup Brown Sugar
- 1/2 Cup + 1 Tbsp Butter, Unsalted
- 1/3 Cup Cocoa Powder, Dark And Unsweetened
- 2 Eggs, Beaten
- 1 1/2 Cups Flour, All-Purpose
- 1/3 Cup Miniature Chocolate Chips
- 2 Cups Peanut Butter Chips, Divided
- 1/4 Tsp Sea Salt
- 1/2 Cup Sugar, Granulated
- 1 Tsp Vanilla Extract

Directions:

1. Fire up your Pit Boss Griddle and preheat to medium-low heat. If using a gas or charcoal grill, preheat a cast iron skillet.
2. In a mixing bowl, whisk together the flour, cocoa powder, baking soda, and salt. Set aside.
3. Set a metal saucepan on the griddle, then add ½ cup of butter to melt. Whisk in the sugars and vanilla extract and cook for 2 minutes. Remove the pan from the griddle, and transfer contents to a large mixing bowl.
4. Slowly pour the beaten eggs into the sugar mixture, whisking constantly to temper the eggs.
5. Add the dry mixture to the wet ingredients until just combined. Fold in 1 cup of peanut butter chips and chocolate chips. Refrigerate mixture for 15 to 30 minutes.
6. Remove the dough from the refrigerator, then add an additional cup of peanut butter chips.
7. Portion dough into 16 to 18 cookie balls.
8. Melt 1 tablespoon of butter on the griddle, then transfer the cookie balls to the griddle. Press down gently on the cookies, then cook for 10 to 12 minutes, flipping halfway.
9. Transfer cookies to a cooling rack for 5 minutes before enjoying.

Bananas Foster

Servings: 4
Cooking Time: 10 Minutes
Ingredients:
- 1/3 Cup Banana Nectar
- 4 Bananas, Quartered
- 3/4 Cup Brown Sugar
- 1/4 Cup Butter
- 1/2 Tsp Cinnamon, Ground
- 1/3 Cup Dark Rum
- Vanilla Ice Cream

Directions:

1. Fire up your Pit Boss Griddle and preheat to medium heat. If using a gas or charcoal grill, preheat a cast iron skillet.
2. Place a large skillet on the griddle, then melt butter in the skillet. Whisk in brown sugar and cinnamon, stirring until sugar dissolves.
3. Add the banana nectar and bananas. Stir to coat
4. Once the bananas begin to soften and turn brown, add the rum. Stir, then ignite the sauce with a stick lighter. After the flames subside, simmer the sauce for 2 minutes.
5. Divide the bananas among 4 scoops/bowls of vanilla ice cream, then spoon the warm sauce over the top of the ice cream. Serve immediately.

How To Make Sourdough Bread

Servings: 4
Cooking Time: 45 Minutes
Ingredients:
- 200 G All-Purpose Flour
- 200 G Bread Flour
- 10 G Kosher Salt
- 80 G Sourdough Starter
- 350 G Water, Bottled, Room Temp
- 50 G Whole Wheat Flour

Directions:

1. Day 1: Use a kitchen scale to weigh out 25 grams whole wheat flour, 25 grams all-purpose flour, and 50 grams of bottled water. Place flour in a glass jar with a lid, then pour water on top. Stir with a fork to combine. The mixture should resemble thick paste. Cover the jar and place it in a warm location, ideally 70°F, for 24 hours.
2. Day 2: Use a kitchen scale to weigh out 25 grams whole wheat flour, 25 grams all-purpose flour, and 50 grams of bottled water. Discard half of the starter and add the weighed ingredients to the jar. Stir with a fork to combine. Cover the jar and place it in a warm location for 24 hours.

3. Day 3: You will likely see a few more bubbles today. Use a kitchen scale to weigh out 25 grams whole wheat flour, 25 grams all-purpose flour, and 50 grams of bottled water. Discard half of the starter and add the weighed ingredients to the jar. Stir with a fork to combine. Cover the jar and place it in a warm location for 24 hours.

4. Day 4: You should see a lot more bubbles and the starter should increase in volume. Use a kitchen scale to weigh out 25 grams whole wheat flour, 25 grams all-purpose flour, and 50 grams of bottled water. Stir with a fork to combine. Cover the jar and place it in a warm location for 24 hours.

5. Day 5: The starter will be very bubbly and double in volume. This starter is now ready to use! Use the starter or refrigerate for up to 4 days, then feed again.

Lemon Chicken, Broccoli & String Beans Foil Packs

Servings: 4
Cooking Time: 20 Minutes
Ingredients:

- 2 Cups Broccoli
- 3 Tbsp Butter, Melted
- 4 Chicken, Boneless/Skinless
- 1 Garlic, Minced
- 1 1/2 Tsp Italian Seasoning, Dried
- 1 Lemon, Sliced
- Pepper
- Salt
- 1 Cup String Beans

Directions:

1. Start your grill on smoke with the lid open until a fire is established in the burn pot (3-7 minutes). Preheat to 450F.

2. Lay four 12 x 12 inch pieces of foil out on a flat surface, then place one chicken breast in the middle of each foil.

3. Divide the broccoli and string beans between the four foil packs. Thinly slice the lemon, split them between each foil pack, and place the slices on, in and around the chicken and vegetables.

4. Mix the butter, garlic, juice of the remaining lemon, and Italian seasoning together, and then brush over the chicken and vegetables. Sprinkle with salt and pepper to taste.

5. Fold the foil over the chicken and vegetables to close the pack, and pinch the ends together so the pack will remain closed.

6. Grill for 7-9 minutes on each side. Turn o grill, remove the foil packets, and serve immediately.

Smoked Lemon Sweet Tea

Servings: 6 - 8
Cooking Time: 60 Minutes
Ingredients:

- 8 Black Tea Bags
- 4 Cups Boiling Water
- 2 Cups Ice
- 8 Lemons
- 2 Cups Sugar
- 2 Cups Water

Directions:

1. Place the tea bags in a heat-safe pitcher. Bring 4 Cups of water to a boil and pour over tea bags. Let steep for 5-10 minutes. Remove tea bags and set pitcher aside to cool.

2. Turn on your Pit Boss and set to smoke mode. Combine 2 cups of sugar and 2 cup water in a small aluminum pan. Smoke fo about 45 minutes, stirring occasionally, o until the mixture reduces to a thick, simp syrup. Remove from the grill and let it co

3. Fire up your Pit Boss to 450°F and open the flame broiler. If using a charcoal or gas grill, set heat to high.

4. Cut the lemons in half and sear over the flame broiler until charred, about 7 minutes. Remove from grill and set aside to cool.

5. Juice the lemons into a medium bowl. Pour lemon juice through a metal strainer into the tea pitcher to remove seeds and pulp.

6. Pour the cooled simple syrup into pitcher and stir until fully incorporated with tea and lemons. Add 2 cups of ice and refrigerate until serving.

Pancake Casserole

Servings: 6
Cooking Time: 60 Minutes
Ingredients:
- 2 Tbsp Butter
- 1/2 Cup Chocolate Chips
- 4 Egg
- Maple Syrup
- 12 - 14 Pancakes
- Powdered Sugar
- 1/4 Cup Sugar, Granulated
- 1 Tsp Vanilla Extract
- 1 1/2 Cup Whole Milk

Directions:
1. In a mixing bowl, whisk together flour, baking powder, sugar, and salt. Then pour in the milk, egg and melted butter; mix until smooth.

2. Fire up your Pit Boss Platinum Series KC Combo and preheat the griddle to medium-low flame. If using a gas or charcoal grill, preheat a large cast iron skillet over medium-low heat.

3. Lightly oil the griddle, then scoop the batter onto the griddle, using approximately ¼ cup for each pancake. Cook 1 to 2 minutes per side, until golden

brown. Set aside to cool for 15 minutes, then assemble the casserole.

Double Stuffed Sweet Potatoes

Servings: 6
Cooking Time: 45 Minutes
Ingredients:
- 2 Bacon, Strip
- 1/4 Cup Green Onion
- 2 Potato, Sweet
- 1 Cup Shredded Cheddar Cheese

Directions:
1. Prepare to stuff yourself with Double Stuffed Sweet Potatoes.

2. Fill the hopper with your desired blend of hardwood pellets and preheat your grill to 400°F with the flame broiler fully closed. Bake the sweet potatoes for 30 minutes or until soft.

3. Remove potatoes from the grill and cut them in half (lengthwise). Next, scoop out the potato into a mixing bowl. Using a fork or electric mixer, diligently mash the potato and return it home to the skins. Load the tops with green onion, bacon and cheese.

4. Return the newly loaded skins to the grill for 10 minutes or until the cheese has melted. Garnish with salt, pepper and sour cream for an appetizer that will surely morph into a full meal.

Mexican Cornbread Casserole

Servings: 6
Cooking Time: 30 Minutes
Ingredients:

- 1 Lb Beef, Ground
- 1 15Oz Drained Black Beans, Can
- 1 Box Corn Muffin Mix
- 1 15Oz Enchilada Sauce, Can
- 1 Onion, Chopped
- 1 15Oz Drained Pinto Beans, Can

Directions:

1. Start Grill at 300 degrees with flame broiler open.
2. Mix corn muffin mix according to directions.
3. Place cast iron skillet over flame broiler and heat for a few minutes, leaving Grill lid open.
4. Add onion and ground beef/sausage to skillet and break up
5. Cook until meat is done about 5 to 10 minutes.
6. Add both cans of beans, and enchilada sauce, stir to combine.
7. Bring mixture to a simmer.
8. Carefully close flame broiler and turn Grill up to 400 degrees.
9. Spread prepared corn muffin mix over top of meat and bean mixture and bake for 15 minutes until cornbread mixture is lightly browned.
10. Let sit 15 minutes before serving.

Basic Crescent Rolls

Servings: 8
Cooking Time: 12 Minutes
Ingredients:

- 1 Crescent Dough, Can

Directions:

1. Preheat your Grill to 375F.
2. Unroll the dough and separate into triangles. Roll up the triangles and place on an ungreased nonstick cookie sheet.

Bake for 10 -12 minutes on your Grill. You will know that they are finished when the rolls are golden brown.

Thanksgiving Smoked Turkey

Servings: 6 - 8
Cooking Time: 300 Minutes
Ingredients:

- 1 Turkey Brining Kits
- 12 – 14 Lbs Turkey
- 1 Gallon Water, Cold
- 4 Cups + 1 Gallon Water, Warm

Directions:

1. Start by defrosting the turkey overnight in the refrigerator.
2. Once turkey has been defrosted begin to make the brine by adding 4 cups of water and the brine mixture to a large stockpot.
3. Bring the mixture to a boil and add 1 gallon of cold water.
4. Place the turkey in the brine bag and pour the brine mixture over the turkey and refrigerate 1 hour per pound.
5. Once turkey has been brined rinse the turkey with cold water and set on a pan.
6. Using the seasoning in the brine box, season the turkey. Once turkey has been seasoned start your Pit Boss smoker by turning it to 275 degrees.
7. Place your turkey in the smoker and place the temperature probe in the deepest part of the breast. Cook at 275 until the breast and thigh meat internal temperature has reached 165°F to 170°F.
8. Remove the turkey from the smoker, let cool, and cut the turkey into your desired pieces. Enjoy!

Mint Chocolate Chip Cookies

Servings: 24

Cooking Time: 12 Minutes

Ingredients:

- 1/2 Cup Butter, Melted
- 1 Package Chocolate Chip Cookie Mix
- 8-10 Drop Food Coloring
- 1/2 Tsp Mint, Extract

Directions:

1. Preheat your Grill at 350F.
2. Follow the directions on the back of the Chocolate Chip Cookie mix and also add the mint extract and green food coloring. Mix until combined.
3. On a baking sheet lined with parchment paper, drop balls of dough about 2 tbsp in size onto the pan.
4. Place in your Grill and bake for 10-12 minutes. Let cool for a couple minutes before removing from the pan. Enjoy!

Five Cheese Mac And Cheese By Chef Shaun O'neale

Servings: 6 - 10

Cooking Time: 60 Minutes

Ingredients:

- 5 Tbsp All-Purpose Flour
- 4 Strips Bacon
- Black Pepper
- 2 Cups Breadcrumbs
- 4 Oz Brie
- 4 Oz Brie Cheese
- ½ Cup Butter, Melted
- 12 Oz Cheddar Cheese, Grated
- 3 Cloves Garlic, Minced
- 2 Tbsp Extra Virgin Olive Oil
- 1 Tsp Fresh Grated Nutmeg
- 1 Tsp Ground Cayenne
- 8 Oz, Grated Gruyere Cheese
- 1 Cup Heavy Cream
- 1, Minced Jalapeno Pepper
- 4 Oz Mozzarella Cheese, Grated
- 2 Tbsp Parsley, Minced Fresh
- 12 Oz Raclette
- To Taste Salt
- 5 Tbsp Unsalted Butter
- 4 Oz Whole Milk, Warm
- 1 Yellow Onion, Diced

Directions:

1. Heat your Pit Boss Pellet Grill to 350 degrees with the heat shield closed. Bring a large saucepan of water to a boil. Add the pasta and cook according to the package instructions for al dente. Drain.
2. Heat the oil in a large saucepan over medium-high heat.
3. Add the onion and cook for about 5 minutes, stirring often, until lightly colored, then add the garlic and the jalapeño and cook for 2 more minutes.
4. Reduce the heat to medium, add the butter, and stir until melted. Add the flour and cook, stirring often, for 5 minutes to form a light roux.
5. Add the cheeses, the milk, and cream, reduce the heat to medium-low, and cook, stirring often, until the cheese is melted, and a smooth sauce comes together, about 7 minutes.
6. Stir in the cayenne and truffle oil, then add the pasta and stir to fully coat it in the sauce. Season with salt and pepper. Transfer the mixture to a 12-inch cast-iron skillet and cover with aluminum foil.
7. Place on the grill and bake for 20 minutes. Remove the foil and cover the mac and cheese with the breadcrumbs.
8. Return to the grill and bake for another 15 to 20 minutes, until the cheese is bubbling and the breadcrumbs are golden brown. Serve family style right out of the skillet.

Crack Cake With Smoked Berry Sauce

Servings: 12
Cooking Time: 90 Minutes
Ingredients:

- 12 Oz Blackberries
- 18 Oz Blueberries, Fresh
- 1/4 Cup Brown Sugar
- 2 Tsp Cinnamon, Ground
- 4 Eggs
- 2 Tbsp Flour
- 1 3/4 Cup Granulated Sugar
- 1 Lemon, Juice & Zest
- 1/2 Cup Unsalted Butter
- 3.4 Ounce Box Vanilla Instant Pudding Mix
- 3/4 Cup Vegetable Oil
- 3/4 Cup Water
- 1 Cup White Wine
- 1 Box Yellow Cake Mix

Directions:

1. Fire up your Pit Boss Platinum Series Lockhart Grill and set to Smoke mode. If using a gas or charcoal grill, set it up for low, indirect heat.
2. Place blueberries and blackberries on a sheet tray, then transfer to upper shelf of smoking cabinet. Make sure that the sear slide and side dampers are open, then increase temperature to 375°F, to ensure the cabinet maintains temperature between 225° F and 250° F. Smoke for 30 to 45 minutes.
3. Place cast iron skillet on grill grate. Add sugar, lemon juice and zest, and wine to skillet. Stir with a wooden spoon until sugar dissolves, then add berries from smoking cabinet.
4. Simmer berries for 15 minutes, then remove sauce from grill to cool.
5. While berries are smoking, prepare cake pans and batter. Grease and flour 2 - 9-inch round cake pans. Set aside.

6. In a large mixing bowl, combine cake mix brown sugar, granulated sugar, pudding mix, cinnamon, eggs, water, oil, and white wine. Using a hand mixer, mix on low speed for 1 minute, then slowly increase mixing speed to high, and beat an additional 2 to 3 minutes, or until batter i smooth.
7. Evenly distribute batter among cake pans then place pans on grill shelf and bake at 350° F, for 25 to 30 minutes, or until a toothpick inserted comes out clean. Remove from grill and set aside to cool slightly.
8. While cake is cooling, prepare glaze. Melt butter with sugar in a sauce pot on the gri Stir for 3 minutes, then add wine. Remov from grill and set aside.
9. Turn out cake onto a sheet tray lined with parchment. Use a toothpick to poke holes in the cake, then slowly pour hot glaze over cake.
10. Spread half of smoked berry sauce on top of one layer, then place second cake layer on top. Pour additional sauce on top of cake and dust with powdered sugar, if desired. Serve warm, or room temperatu

Cheesy Potato Casserole

Servings: 15
Cooking Time: 105 Minutes
Ingredients:

- 1 Cream Of Celery Soup, Can
- 1 Family Size Cream Of Mushroom Soup, Can
- Pan Spray
- 1 - 10 Oz Pic Sweet Frozen Seasoning Blend
- Pit Boss Steak Seasoning
- 1 - 32 Oz Bag Potato, Frozen Cubes
- 8 Oz Sour Cream
- 1 Lb Cubbed Valveeta Cheese Sauce

Directions:

1. Start Grill at 350 degrees
2. Spray foil pan with pan spray
3. Place all ingredients into mixing bowl except potatoes and mix well
4. Place potatoes into mixing bowl with mixture and mix well.
5. Empty potatoes into foil pan.
6. Cover with aluminum foil and bake at 350 for 1 hour.
7. Remove foil and stir thoroughly, bake for 30 minutes more or until bubbly
8. Let rest at least 15 minutes before serving.

Monster Cookies

Servings: 20
Cooking Time: 35 Minutes
Ingredients:
- 2 Packages Candy Eyeballs
- Green, Blue And Purple Food Coloring
- 1 Box Of Yellow Gluten Free Cake Mix
- 1/2 Cup (Optional) Granulated Sugar
- 2 Large Eggs
- 1/3 Cup Powdered Sugar
- 1 Teaspoon Pure Vanilla Extract
- 6 Tablespoon Melted Vegan Butter (Unsalted)

Directions:
1. Preheat your grill to 350°F. Close the flame broiler.
2. Line two large baking sheets with parchment paper. In a large bowl, combine cake mix, melted butter, eggs (or egg substitute), powdered sugar, sugar (optional), and vanilla and stir until combined. (substitute 2 flax eggs for Vegan – 1 tbsp flaxseed meal and 5 tbsp water per egg).
3. Divide dough between 3 bowls and dye each bowl a different color.(We used green, blue and purple).
4. Roll dough into tablespoon-sized balls.
5. Place about 2" apart on the baking sheet and grill until tops have cracked and the tops look set, 8 to 10 minutes. – Turn half way through baking, after 4-5 minutes.
6. Immediately, while the cookies are still warm, stick candy eyeballs all over the cookies.
7. Let cool completely before serving.

Cheesecake Skillet Brownie

Servings: 2
Cooking Time: 30 Minutes
Ingredients:
- 1 Box Brownie Mix
- 1 Package Cream Cheese
- 2 Egg
- 1/2 Cup Oil
- 1 Can Pie Filling, Blueberry
- 1/2 Cup Sugar
- 1 Tsp Vanilla
- 1/4 Cup Water, Warm

Directions:
1. Combine all brownie ingredients and mix. In a separate bowl, combine cream cheese, sugar, egg and vanilla and mix until smooth. Grease skillets and pour in brownie batter. Top with cheesecake and cherry pie filling, using a knife to blend to give it that marbled look.
2. Place in your Grill at 350F and bake for about 30 minutes.
3. Let cool for about 10 minutes and enjoy!

Peanut Butter Cookies

Servings: 24
Cooking Time: 15 Minutes

Ingredients:

- 1 Egg
- 1 Cup Peanut Butter
- 1 Cup Sugar

Directions:

1. Start your Grill on smoke with the lid open until a fire is established in the burn pot (3-7 minutes). Preheat to HIGH. Combine all ingredients in a bowl. Drop tablespoon amounts of dough on a prepared baking sheet and bake in your Grill for 15-20 minutes. Allow cookies to cool for 5 minutes on the baking sheet before you enjoy!

Bbq Chicken Pizza On The Grill

Servings: 4
Cooking Time: 10 Minutes

Ingredients:

- 3 Boneless, Skinless Chicken Breast
- 5 Cups Flour, Strong
- 3 Cups Georgia Style Bbq Sauce
- 3 Cups Mozzarella Cheese, Shredded
- 1 Tsp Olive Oil
- 3 Cups Pit Boss Georgia Style Bbq Sauce
- 1 1/2 Cups Red Bell Peppers, Diced
- 1 1/2 Cups Red Onion, Diced
- 1 Tsp Sugar
- 1/2 Cup Water, Hot
- 1 1/4 Cup Water, Warm
- 2 Tsb Active Yeast, Instant

Directions:

1. Roll your pizza dough so it forms a base about a 1/2 inch thick. To impress your friends and family, you'll want to aim for a nice, pizza like shape. HINT: use a sprinkle of cornmeal on the countertop to aid in moving the dough.

2. Now for the toppings! Start by spreading 1 cup of Georgia Style BBQ sauce onto each base. Make sure to leave a small portion for the crust! Next, load up with sliced, cooked chicken breasts, diced red onions and red bell peppers before finishing off with a two cups of shredded mozzarella cheese.

3. Place the pizza stone in your grill and preheat to 500°F. Pick up your pizza using a flat surface like a chopping board and slide the pizza carefully onto the hot stone Close the lid and let your homemade wood-fired pizza bake for 10 - 12 minutes. Remove once your pizza has a golden crust and the cheese is bubbling. Cut and serve for pizza you'll hardly want to share.

Loaded Portobello Mushrooms

Servings: 4
Cooking Time: 20 Minutes

Ingredients:

- 8 Bacon, Strip
- 1 Cup Cheddar Cheese, Shredded
- 3 Cloves Garlic, Minced
- Green Onion
- 4 Large Portobello Mushrooms

Directions:

1. Preheat your Grill to 350 degrees F.
2. Core the mushrooms and remove the gills completely.
3. Sprinkle garlic in each mushroom, followed by bacon, 1/4 cup cheese, more bacon and lastly green onions.
4. Place on the grates of your Grill and cook for about 20 minutes.
5. Serve hot. Be careful taking the first bite - they"re very juicy! Enjoy!

Homemade Blueberry Pancakes

Servings: 4
Cooking Time: 10 Minutes
Ingredients:

- 2 Cups Blueberries, Fresh
- 1 Cup Pancake Mix
- 1/2 Cup Sugar
- 3/4 Cup Water, Warm

Directions:

1. Preheat your Grill to 350°F. Place the cast iron griddle on the grates of your grill.
2. In a large bowl, pour water, pancake mix and 1/2 cup of the blueberries and mix until combined.
3. Pour the batter onto the griddle in 4 equal parts. Cook with the lid closed for about 6 minutes, or until the edges of the pancakes are slightly cooked. Flip each pancake and continue cooking for another 4 minutes.
4. Pour the hot blueberry sauce over your freshly cooked pancakes and enjoy!

Lemon Pepper Chicken Wings

Servings: 4
Cooking Time: 30 Minutes
Ingredients:

- 1/4 Cup Black Peppercorns, Ground
- 4 Pounds Chicken, Wing
- 2 Tsp Coriander, Ground
- 2 Tsp Garlic Powder
- 2-3 Tbsp Lemon, Zest
- 1 Tsp Salt, Kosher
- 3 Tsp Dried Thyme, Fresh Sprigs

Directions:

1. Start your Grill on "smoke" with the lid open until a fire is established in the burn pot (3-7 minutes). Preheat to 400F.
2. In a bowl, begin to mix the ground pepper and zest of the lemon together, then add the rest of the ingredients.
3. Place the wings in a bowl and toss with a little olive oil, add a few tablespoons of the seasoning, toss with your hands, then

repeat until the wings are well seasoned to your liking.
4. Place the wings on the grill, and cook them for about 15 minutes, then flip and grill for another 15 minutes.
5. Continue to flip the wings, until they are done and crispy. Remove the wings from the grill, and serve.

Strawberry Rhubarb Pie

Servings: 8
Cooking Time: 30 Minutes
Ingredients:

- 1/3 Cup Flour
- 1 Tbsp Lemon, Zest
- 1 Prepard Pie Shell, Deep
- 3 Stalks Rhubarb
- 2 1/2 Cups Strawberry
- 1 Cup Sugar

Directions:

1. Summer baking never has to stop when you can use your Wood Pellet Grill to bake anything from cookies to pie! In this recipe, we will show you how to bake a delicious barbecued strawberry rhubarb pie without turning your kitchen into an oven.
2. Preheat grill to 400°F.
3. Slice rhubarb and strawberries into bite sized pieces. Combine sugar, flour and lemon zest with rhubarb and strawberries. Pour into prepared pie crust. Cover with top crust.
4. Bake in Grill for 1 hour or until crust is crispy.
5. Serve hot.

Cheesy Garlic Pull Apart Bread

Servings: 2
Cooking Time: 20 Minutes
Ingredients:

- 1 Loaf Bread, Sourdough Round
- 2 1/2 Tbsp Butter, Salted
- 8 Oz Fontina Cheese
- 1 Grated Garlic, Roasted
- 1/4 Cup Parsley, Minced Fresh
- 1 Tsp Red Flakes Pepper
- 1 Pinch Salt

Directions:

1. Start your Grill on "smoke" with the lid open until a fire is established in the burn pot (3-7 minutes). Preheat to 300F.
2. In a small bowl, add the soft butter, grated garlic, red pepper flakes, sea salt, and ¼ cup of the chopped parsley, and whisk together. With a bread serrated knife, cut 1-inch slices into the bread, not cutting all the way through the bottom of the load. With a butter knife, spread a thin layer of the butter mixture on each slice of the bread. Take the serrated knife again, and cut across the loaf to form 1 inch squares. Next, slice the cheese into small thin slices, then stuff one slice into each bread opening. Place the bread on a baking sheet, and cover tightly with aluminum foil. Place on the grill for about 10 minutes, remove the foil, and grill for a few more minutes until the top is nicely golden and the cheese is oozing. Remove from the grill, sprinkle with fresh parsley leaves, then serve.

Bourbon Bacon Brownies

Servings: 16
Cooking Time: 60 Minutes
Ingredients:

- 2 Cup All-Purpose Flour
- 1/4 Cup Bourbon
- 1 Cup Brown Sugar
- 1 Cup Canola Oil
- Caramel Sauce
- 1.5 Cup Cocoa Powder
- 1 Tablespoon Hickory Honey Sea Salt
- 2 Tablespoon Instant Coffee
- 6 Large Eggs
- 1/2 Teaspoon Pit Boss Smoked Infused Hickory Honey Sea Salt
- 1 Cup Powdered Sugar
- 6 Slices Bacon, Raw
- 4 Tablespoons Water
- 3 Cups White Sugar

Directions:

1. Start up your Pit Boss. Once it's fired up, set the temperature to 400°F.
2. In a large mixing bowl, whisk together the cocoa, powdered sugar, white sugar, instant coffee and flour.
3. To the flour mixture, add the eggs, oil and water until just combined.
4. Spray the 9 x 13 pan well with cooking spray.
5. Pour half the batter in the pan, drizzle with caramel.
6. Pour other half of batter on top and drizzle with caramel again and add candied bacon to the top.
7. Bake the brownies in the smoker for 1 hour, or until a toothpick inserted in the center of the pan comes out clean.
8. Remove from the smoker and allow to cool before slicing.

Bossin' Nachos

Servings: 6
Cooking Time: 10 Minutes
Ingredients:

- 1 Pound Beef, Ground
- 3 Cups Cheddar Cheese, Shredded
- 1 Green Bell Pepper, Diced
- 1/2 Cup Green Onion
- 1/2 Cup Red Onion, Diced
- 1 Large Bag Tortilla Chip

Directions:

1. Start your Grill on "smoke" with the lid open until a fire is established in the burn pot (3-4 minutes). Preheat to 350°F.
2. While you're waiting, empty a large bag of nacho chips evenly onto a cast iron pan. Start loading up with toppings - cooked ground beef, red onion, red pepper, cheese, green onions. These are just the toppings we had on hand, so feel free to add anything you like! Make sure you do a couple layers of chips so everyone gets a good serving of nachos. And don't be skimpy with the cheese - lay it on heavy!
3. Place your loaded nachos on the grill and let the hot smoke melt your toppings into one cheesy creation. Heat at 350°F for 10 minutes or until the cheese has fully melted. Remove and serve with sour-cream and salsa.

Homemade Corn Tortillas

Servings: 11 - 22
Cooking Time: 10 Minutes
Ingredients:

- Cooking Spray
- 10 Oz Masa Harina
- 1 Tbsp Vegetable Oil
- 9 Oz Water, Hot
- 3 Oz Water, Room Temperature

Directions:

1. In a large mixing bowl, mix together masa and hot water. Mix with a wooden spoon or by hand. Cover with plastic wrap and allow to sit at room temperature for 1 hour.
2. Turn out the dough. Dough will be crumbly. Incorporate 1 tablespoon of water at a time, while kneading and pressing together, until a soft, smooth texture is reached. If too sticky, add a dusting of Masa.
3. Divide dough into 1 ounce balls, then spray with cooking spray.
4. Place a piece of parchment paper on a tortilla press. Set a dough ball in the center, then top with another piece of parchment paper. Flatten dough ball with the press, then transfer to a sheet tray. Separate each layer with plastic wrap and spray with cooking spray. Repeat until all dough balls are pressed.

Cherry Cobbler

Servings: 8
Cooking Time: 45 Minutes
Ingredients:

- 1 Tsp Baking Powder
- 3 Tbsp Butter, Melted
- 1 Cup Flour
- Ice Cream, Prepared
- 1/4 Tsp Salt
- 3/4 Cup Sugar
- 1/2 Cup Milk

Directions:

1. Preheat your Grill to 350 degrees F.
2. In a bowl, combine flour, sugar, baking powder, salt and mix to incorporate. Stir in butter and milk and mix until combined. In a cast iron pan, dump in cherry pie filling and pile on the prepared topping to cover.
3. Place in your Grill and bake for about 45 minutes, or until the topping is golden brown.

4. Let cool for a couple minutes and serve with ice cream.

Cranberry Apple Sage Stuffing

Servings: 7
Cooking Time: 45 Minutes
Ingredients:

- 10 Cups Day Old Diced Bread, Sliced Loaf
- 2 1/2 Cups Broth, Chicken
- 1 Cup Butter, Unsalted
- 1 Cup Diced Celery, Cut
- 1 1/2 Cups Fresh Cranberries
- 1 Beaten Egg
- 1 Medium Granny Smith Apple, Peel, Core And Dice
- 2 Tbsp Minced Parsley, Fresh
- 1 Tbsp Minced Rosemary, Fresh
- 2 Tbsp Roughly Chopped Sage
- Salt And Pepper
- 1 Tbsp Minced Thyme
- 2 Cups Diced Yellow Onion, Sliced

Directions:

1. Turn your Pit Boss Pellet Grill to smoke mode, let the fire catch and then set to 350°F to preheat.
2. Melt butter over medium heat. Add onions then celery and cook until onions start to become translucent.
3. In a large bowl, mix together bread, apples, cranberries, cooked onion and celery mixture, and fresh herbs.
4. Add half of the chicken broth to the mixture and stir.
5. Beat together eggs and the rest of the chicken broth in a small bowl. Pour into the bread mixture and stir until completely combined.
6. Add salt and pepper to taste.
7. Pour stuffing into a cast iron pan or baking dish. Cover with foil and bake on the grill for 30 minutes. Remove the foil and cook for an additional 15 minutes.

8. Serve immediately and enjoy!

Whole Roasted Duck

Servings: 5
Cooking Time: 150 Minutes
Ingredients:

- 2 Tbsp Baking Soda
- 1 Tbsp Chinese Five Spice
- 1 Whole Thawed Duck
- 1 Granny Smith Apple, Peel, Core And Dice
- 1 Quartered Orange, Slice
- 2 Tbsp Pit Boss Champion Chicken Seasoning, Divided

Directions:

1. Wash the duck under cold running water, inside and out, then pat dry with paper towel.
2. Mix Champion Chicken seasoning and Chinese Five Spice together. Mix with baking soda for extra crispy skin. Season the duck, inside and out.
3. Tuck the orange and apple slices in the cavity.
4. When you're ready to cook, turn your Pit Boss grill to smoke mode, let the fire catch and then set to 300 degrees F (149 degrees C) to preheat.
5. Add duck to a roasting pan or directly onto the grill grate.
6. Roast for 2 – 2 ½ hours or until the skin is brown and crispy and the internal temperature of the thigh is 160 degrees F (71 degrees C).
7. Add foil loosely over the duck and let rest for 15 minutes.

Double Chocolate Cake

Servings: 12
Cooking Time: 40 Minutes
Ingredients:

- 1 1/2 Tsp Baking Soda

- 1/2 Cup Butter, Melted
- 1 Cup Buttermilk, Low Fat
- 1 Jar Chocolate Icing, Prepared
- 3/4 Cup Cocoa, Powder
- 1 Cup Coffee, Hot
- 2 Large Egg
- 1 3/4 Cups Flour, All-Purpose
- 3/4 Tsp Salt
- 2 Cups Sugar
- 1 Tbsp Vanilla

Directions:

1. Preheat your to 350 degrees F.
2. Stir together flour, sugar, cocoa, baking soda and salt in a large bowl. Combine eggs, buttermilk, butter and coffee and mix until smooth. Add in hot coffee and stir until combined and the dough is runny.
3. Pour the batter into two prepared baking pans and bake on the top rack of your for 40 minutes, turning the pans 180 degrees halfway through.
4. Allow to cool and then frost with chocolate icing.

Margherita Pizza

Servings: 6
Cooking Time: 25 Minutes
Ingredients:

- Basil, Chopped
- 2 Cups Flour, All-Purpose
- Mozzarella Cheese, Sliced Rounds
- 1 Cup Pizza Sauce
- 1 Teaspoon Salt
- 1 Teaspoon Sugar
- 1 Tomato, Sliced
- 1 Cup Water, Warm
- 1 Teaspoon Yeast, Instant

Directions:

1. Combine the water, yeast, and sugar in a small bowl and let sit for about 5 minutes.
2. In a large bowl, stir together the flour and salt. Pour in the yeast mixture and mix

until a soft dough forms. Knead for about 2 minutes. Place in an oiled bowl and cover with a cloth. Let the dough sit and rise for about 45 minutes or until the dough has doubled in size.

3. Roll out on a flat, floured surface (or on a pizza stone) until you"ve reached your desired shape and thickness.
4. Preheat your Grill to 350 degrees F.
5. On the rolled out dough, pour on the pizza sauce, cheese, and then tomatoes and basil. Place in your Grill and bake for about 25 minutes, or until the cheese is melted and slightly golden brown.

Smoked Beer Cheese Dip

Servings: 6
Cooking Time: 20 Minutes
Ingredients:

- 6 Oz Beer, Can
- 8 Oz Cream Cheese
- 1 Tsp Onion Powder
- ½ Tsp Pepper
- ½ Tsp Salt
- 2 Cups Shredded Cheese

Directions:

1. Fire up your Pit Boss Grill and set the temperature to 350°F. If you're using a gas or charcoal grill, set it up for medium high heat. Preheat with lid closed for 10-15 minutes.
2. In the cast iron pan add cream cheese, shredded cheese, beer, onion powder, salt and pepper. Once grill is at 350°F place cast iron skillet onto the grill and cook for about 10 minutes, stir and cook for another 5-10 minutes.
3. Top with more shredded cheese and fresh parsley. Serve with fresh baked pretzels as well.

Chili Fries

Servings: 6
Cooking Time: 10 Minutes

Ingredients:

- 1 Cup Cheddar Cheese, Shredded
- 1 Cup Chili Con Carne, Prepared
- 1 Bag French Fries
- 1 Tablespoon Olive Oil
- 1 Tablespoon Sweet Heat Rub

Directions:

1. Set up your Pit Boss. Once it's fired up, set the temperature to 350°F. If you're using charcoal or gas, set it up for medium high heat.
2. Bake the fries according to manufacturer's instructions. Once the fries are done, place them in a large bowl and add the olive oil and Sweet Heat Rub. Toss the fries to coat. Once everything is well coated with the oil and seasoning, spread the fries on a baking sheet.
3. Top the fries with the chili and the shredded cheddar cheese. Place the baking sheet on the grill and grill for 7-10 minutes, or until the cheese is melted and bubbly, and the chili is warm all the way through.
4. Remove the baking sheet from the grill and serve the fries immediately.

Pit Boss Chicken Pot Pie

Servings: 6
Cooking Time: 60 Minutes

Ingredients:

- 2 Chicken, Boneless/Skinless
- 1 Cream Of Chicken Soup, Can
- 1 Tsp Curry Powder
- 1/2 Cup Mayo
- 1 1/2 Cups Mixed Frozen Vegetables
- 1 Onion, Sliced
- 2 Frozen Pie Shell, Deep
- 1/2 Cup Sour Cream

Directions:

1. Start your Grill on "smoke" with the lid open until a fire is established in the burn pot (3-4 minutes). Preheat to 425F.
2. Cut the onion in half and place on the grates of the grill. If you"re using fresh chicken breasts, barbecue the chicken at the same time as the onions. The chicken is fully cooked when the internal temperature reached 170F. While the onion and chicken are cooking, prepare the pie crust by putting one crust in a pie plate. When the chicken and onions are done, shred chicken and chop onion into small pieces and place in the prepared pie plate along with the mixed vegetables.
3. Combine cream of chicken soup, mayo, sour cream, and curry powder in a bowl. Pour into the pie crust with the chicken and mix to combine. Wet the sides of the bottom crust with a small amount of water and top with the second pie crust. Push gently along the sides of the crust to seal the two pie crusts together.
4. Place in the and bake for 40 minutes, or until the crust is golden brown. Serve hot

SEAFOOD RECIPES

Seared Ahi Tuna Steak

Servings: 2
Cooking Time: 60 Minutes

Ingredients:

- 1/2 Cup Gluten Free Soy Sauce
- 1 Large Sushi Grade Ahi Tuna Steak, Patted Dry
- 1/4 Cup Lime Juice
- 2 Tablespoons Rice Wine Vinegar
- 2 Tablespoons Sesame Oil, Divided
- 2 Tablespoons Sriracha Sauce
- 4 Tablespoons Sweet Heat Rub
- 2 Cups Water

Directions:

1. Start up your Pit Boss. Once it's fired up, set the temperature to 400°F. If using gas or charcoal, set it up for high heat over direct heat.
2. In the glass baking dish, pour in the water, soy sauce, lime juice, rice wine vinegar, 1 tablespoon sesame oil, sriracha sauce, and mirin. Whisk the marinade together with the whisk until everything is well combine. Place the ahi steak into the marinade and place the glass baking dish with the ahi steak in the refrigerator for 30 minutes. After 30 minutes, flip the ahi steak over so that the ahi has the chance to fully marinate on all sides, and allow to marinate for 30 more minutes.
3. After the tuna steak has finished marinating, drain off the marinade and pat the steak dry with paper towels on all sides. Pour the Sweet Heat Rub onto the plate and rub the remaining tablespoon of sesame oil generously on all sides of the tuna steak, and then gently place the tuna steak into the seasoning on the plate, turning on all sides to coat evenly.
4. Insert a temperature probe into the thickest part of the ahi steak and place the steak on the hottest part of the grill. Grill the ahi tuna steak for 45 seconds on each side, or just until the outside is opaque and has grill marks. Flip the steak and allow it to grill for another 45 seconds until the outside is just cooked through. The ahi tuna steak's internal temperature should be just at 115°F.
5. Remove the steak from the grill once it reaches 115°F, and immediately slice and serve. The inside of the steak should still be cool and ruby pink.

Crab Stuffed Mushrooms

Servings: 4-6
Cooking Time: 15 Minutes

Ingredients:

- 1 Package Cream Cheese, Softened
- 1/2 (2 Oz) Package Imitation Crab, Chopped
- 1 Tablespoon Lemon, Juice
- 2 Teaspoon Lemon, Zest
- 3/4 Cup Panko Japanese Bread Crumbs
- 1/2 Cup Divided Parmesan Cheese, Shredded
- 2 Tablespoon Parsley, Fresh
- 1 Teaspoon Pit Boss Chop House Steak Rub
- 12 Porcini Mushroom Caps, Cleaned And Destemmed

Directions:

1. In a large bowl, combine the cream cheese, imitation crab, breadcrumbs, ¼ cup of the parmesan cheese, lemon zest, lemon juice, parsley and Pit Boss Chophouse Steak seasoning. Mix until completely combined.
2. Using a spoon, stuff a large rounded tablespoon of the filling into the mushroom caps and gently pack it into the mushroom. Once all the mushrooms are stuffed, top with the remaining ¼ cup of parmesan cheese.
3. Preheat your Pit Boss grill to 350F. Place the mushrooms onto a grill basket and

grill for 5 minutes until the cheese is bubbly and golden and the mushrooms are tender.

4. Serve while hot and enjoy!

Scallops Wrapped In Bacon

Servings: 4
Cooking Time: 20 Minutes
Ingredients:

- 3 Tbsp Lemon, Juice
- Pepper
- 12 Scallop

Directions:

1. Start your grill on smoke with the lid open until a fire is established in the burn pot (3-7 minutes).
2. Preheat to 400F.Cut the bacon rashers in half, wrap each half around a scallop and use a toothpick to keep it in place.
3. Next drizzle the lemon juice over the scallops, and then place them on a baking tray.
4. Place in the grill, and grill for about 15-20 minutes, or until the bacon is crisp, remove from the grill, then serve.

Shrimp Scampi

Servings: 3
Cooking Time: 10 Minutes
Ingredients:

- 2 Tsp Blackened Sriracha Rub Seasoning
- 1/2 Cup Butter, Cubed, Divided
- 1/2 Tsp Chili Pepper Flakes
- 3 Garlic Cloves, Minced
- To Taste, Lemon Wedges, For Serving
- 1 Lemon, Juice & Zest
- Linguine, Cooked
- 3 Tbsp Parsley, Chopped
- 1 1/2 Lbs Shrimp, Peeled & Deveined
- Toasted Baguette, For Serving

Directions:

1. Fire up your Pit Boss griddle and preheat to medium-high flame. If using a gas or charcoal grill, set it up for medium-high heat.
2. Add half of the butter to the griddle, then sauté the garlic, Blackened Sriracha, and chili flakes for 1 minute, until fragrant.
3. Add the shrimp, turning occasionally for 2 minutes, until opaque.
4. Add the remaining butter, parsley, lemon zest and juice. Toss the shrimp to coat in lemon butter, then remove from the griddle, and transfer to a serving bowl.
5. Serve immediately, with fresh lemon wedges, and toasted baguette. Serve over linguine, spaghetti or zucchini noodles, if desired.

Honey-soy Glazed Salmon

Servings: 4
Cooking Time: 6 Minutes
Ingredients:

- 1 Tsp Chili Paste
- Chives, Chopped
- 2 Grate Garlic, Cloves
- 2 Tbsp Minced Ginger, Fresh
- 1 Tsp Honey
- 2 Tbsp Lemon, Juice
- 4 Salmon, Fillets (Skin Removed)
- 1 Tsp Sesame Oil
- 2 Tbsp Soy Sauce, Low Sodium

Directions:

1. Start your grill on smoke with the lid open until a fire is established in the burn pot (3-7 minutes). Preheat to 400F.
2. Take the salmon and place it in a large resealable plastic bag, and then top with all remaining ingredients, except the chives. Seal the plastic bag and toss evenly to coat the salmon. Marinade in the refrigerator for 20 minutes.

3. After the salmon has been marinading for 20 minutes, place salmon on a flat pan or right on the grates and grill for about 3 minutes, and then flip and grill on the second side for about 3 minutes. Turn off the Grill, remove the pan from grill, plate, garnish with chives, and enjoy!

Grilled Shrimp With Cajun Dip

Servings: 4
Cooking Time: 15 Minutes
Ingredients:

- 1 Grated Garlic Cloves, Peeled
- 1 Tsp Lemon Juice
- ½ Cup Mayonnaise
- 2 Tbsp Olive Oil
- 1 ½ Tbsp Pit Boss Hickory Bacon Rub
- Scallions
- ½ Lb Shelled And Deveined Shrimp
- 1 Cup Sour Cream

Directions:

1. Fire up your Pit Boss grill and preheat to 350°F. If you're using a gas or charcoal grill, set it to medium heat.
2. In a glass mixing bowl, add mayonnaise, sour cream, Cajun seasoning, garlic, lemon juice, hot sauce, and Hickory Bacon. Whisk together until well combined.
3. Cajun shrimp: In a small bowl, add shrimp, olive oil, Cajun-style seasoning and Hickory Bacon seasoning and toss to combine. Set aside.
4. Transfer dip mixture into cast iron ramekin or small Dutch oven and cover with foil. Place on preheated grill and cook for 10-15 minutes, or until dip begins to bubble along the edges. At the same time, place cast iron pan on grill and add shrimp. Cook for about 3-5 minutes on each side or until shrimp are opaque.
5. Remove dip from grill and top with Cajun shrimp and scallions. Serve warm alongside garlic toast squares and enjoy!

Salmon Cakes And Homemade Tartar Sauce

Servings: 4
Cooking Time: 15 Minutes
Ingredients:

- 1 1/2 Cups Breadcrumb, Dry
- 1/2 Tablespoon Capers, Diced
- 1/4 Cup Dill Pickle Relish
- 2 Eggs
- 1 1/4 Cup Mayonnaise, Divided
- 1 Tablespoon Mustard, Grainy
- 1/2 Tablespoon Olive Oil
- 1/2 Red Pepper, Diced Finely
- 1/2 Tablespoon Pit Boss Sweet Rib Rub
- 1 Cup Cooked Salmon, Flaked

Directions:

1. In a large bowl, mix together the salmon, eggs, ¼ cup mayonnaise, breadcrumbs, red bell pepper, Sweet Rib Rub, and mustard. Allow the mixture to sit for 15 minutes to hydrate the breadcrumbs.
2. Start your Pit Boss on "smoke". Once it's fired up, set the temperature to 350°F.
3. In a small bowl, mix together the remaining mayonnaise, dill pickle relish, and diced capers. Set aside.
4. Place the baking sheet on the grill to preheat. Once the baking sheet is hot, drizzle the olive oil over the pan and drop rounded tablespoons of the salmon mixture onto the sheet pan. Press the mixture down into a flat patty with a spatula. Allow to grill for 3 to 5 minutes, then flip and grill for 1 to 2 more minutes. Remove from the grill and serve with the reserved tartar sauce.

Garlic Shrimp Pesto Bruschetta

Servings: 12
Cooking Time: 15 Minutes
Ingredients:

- 12 Slices Bread, Baguette
- 1/2 Tsp Chili Pepper Flakes
- 1/2 Tsp Garlic Powder
- 4 Cloves Garlic, Minced
- 2 Tbsp Olive Oil
- 1/2 Tsp Paprika, Smoked
- 1/4 Tsp Parsley, Leaves
- Pepper
- Pesto
- Salt
- 12 Shrimp, Jumbo

Directions:

1. Start your Grill on "smoke" with the lid open until a fire is established in the burn pot (3-7 minutes). Preheat to 350F. Place the baguette slices on a baking sheet lined with foil. Stir together the olive oil, and minced garlic, then brush both sides of the baguette slices with the mix. Place the pan inside the grill, and bake for about 10-15 minutes.
2. In a skillet, add a splash of olive oil, shrimp, chili powder, garlic powder, smoked paprika, salt pepper, and grill on medium-high heat for about 5 minutes (until the shrimp is pink). Be sure to stir often. Once pink, remove pan from heat. Once the baguettes are toasted, let them cool for 5 minutes, then spread a layer of pesto onto each one, then top with a shrimp, and serve.

Lemon Smoked Salmon

Servings: 4
Cooking Time: 60 Minutes
Ingredients:

- Dill, Fresh
- 1 Lemon, Sliced
- 1 1/2 - 2 Lbs Salmon, Fresh

Directions:

1. Preheat your Grill to 225°F.
2. Place the salmon on a cedar plank. Lay the lemon slices along the top of the salmon. Smoke in your Grill for about 60 minutes.
3. Top with fresh dill and serve.

Grilled Mango Shrimp

Servings: 4
Cooking Time: 5 Minutes
Ingredients:

- 2 Tablespoon Olive Oil
- 1 Pound Raw Tail-On, Thawed And Deveined Shrimp, Uncooked

Directions:

1. Preheat your Pit Boss Grill to 425F. Rinse shrimp off in sink with cold water. Place in bowl and season generously with Mango Magic seasoning and olive oil. Toss well in bowl.
2. Thread several shrimp onto a skewer, so that they are all just touching each other. Repeat with other skewers and remaining shrimp.
3. Grill shrimp for 2 - 3 minutes on each side or until pink and opaque all the way through. Remove from grill and serve immediately.

Grilled Lobster Tails

Servings: 3
Cooking Time: 10 Minutes
Ingredients:

- Tt Black Pepper
- 3/4 Stick Butter, Room Temp
- 2 Tablespoons Chives, Chopped
- 1 Clove Garlic, Minced
- Lemon, Sliced
- 3 (7-Ounce) Lobster, Tail
- Tt Salt, Kosher

Directions:

1. Start your Grill on "SMOKE" with the lid open until a fire is established in the burn pot (3-7 minutes).
2. Preheat grill to 350°F.
3. Blend butter, chives, minced garlic, and black pepper in a small bowl. Cover with plastic wrap and set aside.
4. Butterfly the tails down the middle of the softer underside of the shell. Don't cut entirely through the center of the meat. Brush the tails with olive oil and season with salt, to your liking.
5. Grill lobsters cut side down about 5 minutes until the shells are bright red in color. Flip the tails over and top with a generous tablespoon of herb butter. Grill for another 4 minutes, or until the lobster meat is an opaque white color.
6. Remove from the grill and serve with more herb butter and lemon wedges.

Blackened Salmon

Servings: 4
Cooking Time: 10 Minutes
Ingredients:

- 1 Tablespoon, Optional Cayenne Pepper
- 2 Cloves Garlic, Minced
- 2 Tablespoons Olive Oil
- 4 Tablespoons Pit Boss Sweet Rib Rub
- 2 Pound Salmon, Fillet, Scaled And Deboned

Directions:

1. Start up your Pit Boss Grill. Once it's fired up, set the temperature to 350°F.
2. Remove the skin from the salmon and discard. Brush the salmon on both sides with olive oil, then rub the salmon fillet with the minced garlic, cayenne pepper and Sweet Rib Rub.
3. Grill the salmon for 5 minutes on one side. Flip the salmon and then grill for another 5 minutes, or until the salmon reaches an internal temperature of 145°F. Remove from the grill and serve.

Cedar Smoked Salmon

Servings: 6
Cooking Time: 60 Minutes
Ingredients:

- 1 Tsp Black Pepper
- 3 Cedar Plank, Untreated
- 1 Tsp Garlic, Minced
- 1/3 Cup Olive Oil
- 1 Tsp Onion, Salt
- 1 Tsp Parsley, Minced Fresh
- 1 1/2 Tbsp Rice Vinegar
- 2 Salmon, Fillets (Skin Removed)
- 1 Tsp Sesame Oil
- 1/3 Cup Soy Sauce

Directions:

1. Soak the cedar planks in warm water for an hour or more.
2. In a bowl, mix together the olive oil, rice vinegar, sesame oil, soy sauce, and minced garlic.
3. Add in the salmon and let it marinate for about 30 minutes.
4. Start your grill on smoke with the lid open until a fire is established in the burn pot (3-7 minutes).
5. Preheat grill to 225°F.

6. Place the planks on the grate. Once the boards start to smoke and crackle a little, it's ready for the fish.
7. Remove the fish from the marinade, season it with the onion powder, parsley and black pepper, then discard the marinade.
8. Place the salmon on the planks and grill until it reaches 140°F internal temperature (start checking temp after the salmon has been on the grill for 30 minutes).
9. Remove from the grill, let it rest for 10 mins, then serve.

Cedar Plank Salmon

Servings: 4
Cooking Time: 20 Minutes
Ingredients:
- 1/4 Cup Brown Sugar
- 1/2 Tablespoon Olive Oil
- Pit Boss Competition Smoked Seasoning
- 4 Salmon Fillets, Skin Off

Directions:
1. Soak the untreated cedar plank in water for 24 hours before grilling. When ready to grill, remove and wipe down.
2. Start up your grill. Then, set the temperature to 350°F.
3. In a small bowl, mix the brown sugar, oil, and Lemon Pepper, Garlic, and Herb seasoning. Rub generously over the salmon fillets.
4. Place the plank over indirect heat, then lay the salmon on the plank and grill for 15-20 minutes, or until the salmon is cooked through and flakes easily with a fork. Remove from the heat and serve immediately.

Mango Thai Shrimp

Servings: 4
Cooking Time: 15 Minutes
Ingredients:
- 2 Tablespoons Brown Sugar
- 2 Tablespoons Pit Boss Mango Magic Seasoning
- 1 Pinch (Optional) Red Pepper Flakes
- 1/2 Tablespoons Rice Wine Vinegar
- 1 Pound Raw Tail-On, Thaw And Deveined Shrimp, Uncooked
- 2 Tablespoons Soy Sauce
- 1 Teaspoon Sriracha Hot Sauce
- 1/2 Cup Sweet Chili Sauce

Directions:
1. Preheat your Pit Boss Grill to 425F. Rinse shrimp off in sink with cold water. Place in bowl and put in all of the ingredients listed above. Let marinade for 2 - 4 hours.
2. Thread several shrimp onto a skewer, so that they are all just touching each other. Repeat with other skewers and remaining shrimp.
3. Grill shrimp for 2 - 3 minutes on each side or until pink and opaque all the way through. Remove from grill and serve immediately.

New England Lobster Rolls

Servings: 4
Cooking Time: 35 Minutes
Ingredients:

- 1/2 Cup Butter
- 4 Hot Dog Bun(S)
- 1 Lemon, Whole
- 4 Lobster, Tail
- 1/4 Cup Mayo
- Pepper

Directions:

1. Start your Grill on "smoke" with the lid open until a fire is established in the burn pot (3-7 minutes). Preheat to 300F.
2. Using kitchen shears, cut the shell of the tail and crack in half so that the meat is exposed. Pour in butter and season with pepper. Place the tails meat side up on the grill and cook until the shell has turned red and the meat is white, about 35 minutes.
3. Remove from the grill and separate the shell from the meat. Place the meat in a bowl with mayo, lemon juice and rind and season with pepper. Stir to combine and evenly distribute into the hot dog buns.

Blackened Catfish

Servings: 4
Cooking Time: 10 Minutes
Ingredients:

- ½ Cup Cajun Seasoning
- ¼ Tsp Cayenne Pepper
- 1 Tsp Granulated Garlic
- 1 Tsp Ground Thyme
- 1 Tsp Onion Powder
- 1 Tsp Ground Oregano
- 1 Tsp Pepper
- 4 (5-Oz.) Skinless Catfish Fillets
- 1 Tbsp Smoked Paprika
- 1 Stick Unsalted Butter

Directions:

1. In a small bowl, combine the Cajun seasoning, smoked paprika, onion powder, granulated garlic, ground oregano, ground thyme, pepper and cayenne pepper.
2. Sprinkle fish with salt and let rest for 20 minutes.
3. Fire up your Pit Boss to 450°F. If you're using a gas or charcoal grill, set it up for medium-high heat. Place cast iron skillet on the grill and let it preheat.
4. While grill is preheating, sprinkle catfish fillets with seasoning mixture, pressing gently to adhere. Add half the butter to preheated cast iron skillet and swirl to coat, add more butter if needed. Place fillets in hot skillet and cook 3-5 minutes or until a dark crust has been formed. Flip and cook an additional 3-5 minutes or until the fish flakes apart when pressed gently with your finger.
5. Remove fish from grill and sprinkle evenly with fresh parsley. Serve with lemon wedges and enjoy!

Fish Tacos

Servings: 12
Cooking Time: 10 Minutes
Ingredients:

- 1 Tsp Black Pepper
- 1/4 Tsp Cayenne Pepper
- 1 1/2 Lbs Cod Fish
- 1/2 Tsp Cumin
- 1 Tsp Garlic Powder
- 1 Tsp Oregano
- 1 1/2 Tsp Paprika, Smoked
- 1/2 Tsp Salt

Directions:

1. Preheat your to 350 degrees.
2. Mix together paprika, garlic powder, oregano, cumin, cayenne, salt and pepper. Sprinkle over cod.

3. Place the cod on your preheated for about 5 minutes per side. Toast tortillas over heat, if desired.
4. Break the cod into pieces, smash the avocado, slice the tomatoes in half and place evenly among the tortillas. Top with red onion, lettuce, jalapenos, sour cream, and cilantro. Spritz with lime juice and enjoy!

Smoked Salmon Dip With Grilled Artichoke And Cheese

Servings: 12
Cooking Time: 270 Minutes
Ingredients:

- 28 Oz Artichoke Hearts, Whole, Canned
- 1/2 Cup Breadcrumbs
- 1/2 Cup Brown Sugar
- 8 Oz Cream Cheese
- 1 Tbsp Garlic Powder
- 1 Cup Italian Cheese Blend, Shredded
- 1/4 Cup Kosher Salt
- 1 Cup Mayonnaise
- 2 Tsp Olive Oil
- 1 Tbsp Onion Powder
- 1/2 Cup Parmesan Cheese
- 2 Tbsp Parsley, Chopped
- Tt Pit Boss Blackened Sriracha Rub
- 1 1/4 Lbs Salmon, Fillet, Scaled And Deboned
- Sour Cream
- 1/2 Tsp White Pepper, Ground

Directions:

1. In a small mixing bowl, whisk together the brown sugar, salt, garlic powder, onion powder, and white pepper. This will make twice the cure needed, so be sure and place the remaining half in a resealable plastic bag and save for smoking fish at a later date.
2. Lay a sheet of plastic wrap on a sheet tray and sprinkle a thin layer of the cure on it.

Place the salmon skin-side down on top of the cure, then sprinkle a couple tablespoons of cure on top. Gently press the cure on top of the salmon flesh, then wrap in plastic wrap.
3. Refrigerate for 8 hours, or overnight.
4. Remove salmon from the refrigerator and wash off the cure in the sink, under cold water.
5. Blot salmon with a paper towel, then set salmon skin side on a wire rack. Dry at room temperature for two hours, or until yellowish shimmer appears on the salmon
6. Fire up your Pit Boss Platinum Series Lockhart to 250°F. If using a gas, charcoal or other grill, set it to low, indirect heat.
7. Place the salmon in the upper cabinet. Smoke for 2 hours, then increase the grill temperature to 350° F to maintain a cabinet temperature of 225°F and smoke another 1 to 2 hours, until salmon reache an internal temperature of 145° F.
8. Remove salmon from the cabinet and set aside to rest for 15 minutes, then flake apart. Reserve ½ cup to top dip after grilling.
9. While the salmon is resting, drain the artichokes, then skewer onto metal skewers (if using wooden skewers, make sure to soak in water for 1 hour prior to grilling, or you can use a grill basket as well).
10. Season with Blackened Sriracha, then set on the grill. Grill for 2 to 3 minutes, until lightly browned.
11. Remove from the grill, cool slightly, then roughly chop. Set aside.
12. In a mixing bowl, combine shredded Italian cheese, grated parmesan, breadcrumbs and parsley. Set aside.
13. Place cream cheese, mayonnaise, and sour cream in a cast iron skillet. Stir frequently with a wooden spoon, for about 5 minutes until the mixture is smooth.

14. Carefully fold in flaked salmon and grilled artichoke hearts, then spread breadcrumb mixture over dip.
15. Drizzle with olive oil, then close the grill lid and bake for 25 to 30 minutes, until dip begins to bubble around the edges, and cheese begins to caramelize on top.
16. Remove dip from the grill, top with reserved salmon and a pinch of parsley. Serve warm with bagel chips, crackers, or crusty bread.

Grilled Spicy Lime Shrimp

Servings: 4
Cooking Time: 10 Minutes
Ingredients:

- 2 Tsp Chili Paste
- 1/2 Tsp Cumin
- 2 Cloves Garlic, Minced
- 1 Large Lime, Juiced
- 1/4 Tsp Paprika, Powder
- 1/4 Tsp Red Flakes Pepper
- 1/2 Tsp Salt

Directions:

1. In a bowl, whisk together the lime juice, olive oil, garlic, chili powder, cumin, paprika, salt, pepper, and red pepper flakes.
2. Then pour it into a resealable bag, add the shrimp, toss the coat, let it marinate for 30 minutes.
3. Start your Grill on "smoke" with the lid open until a fire is established in the burn pot (3-7 minutes). Preheat to 400F.
4. Next place the shrimp on skewers, place on the grill, and grill each side for about two minutes until it's done. One finished, remove the shrimp from the grill and enjoy!

TURKEY RECIPES

Hot Turkey Sandwich

Servings: 4
Cooking Time: 10 Minutes

Ingredients:

- 8 Slices Bread, Sliced
- 1 Cup Gravy, Prepared
- 2 Cups Leftover Turkey, Shredded

Directions:

1. Open the flame broiler of your Grill. Start your grill on "smoke" with the lid open until a fire is established in the burn pot (3-7 minutes). Preheat to 400F.
2. Place the BBQ Grill Mat on the grates of your preheated grill and lay the shredded turkey evenly across the mat to reheat for about 10 minutes.
3. Prepare or reheat the gravy. You"ll want to have the gravy warmed and ready as soon as the turkey is reheated and the bread is toasted.
4. Hold each slice of bread over the flame broiler to toast to your liking.
5. When all of your ingredients are hot, scoop 1/2 cup of the shredded turkey onto a piece of bread, generously cover with gravy and top with another piece of toasted bread. Serve immediately.

Boneless Stuffed Turkey Breast

Servings: 6
Cooking Time: 90 Minutes

Ingredients:

- 1 Bay Leaf
- 1/2 Tsp Black Pepper
- 3 Tbsp Butter, Divided
- 1 Celery Rib, Chopped
- To Taste, Cracked Black Pepper
- 4 Oz Cremini Mushrooms
- 1/2 Cup Dried Cranberries
- 2 Garlic Cloves, Minced
- 1 Package, Approx 2Lbs Honeysuckle White® Turkey Breast, Boneless
- 1/2 Cup Marsala Wine
- 1 Tbsp Olive Oil
- 1 Rosemary Sprigs
- 1/2 Tsp Rubbed Sage
- 1/2 Tsp Salt
- To Taste, Sea Salt
- 6 Oz Stuffing Mix
- 1 1/4 Cup Turkey Stock, Divided
- 1 Yellow Onion, Chopped

Directions:

1. Fire up your Pit Boss Platinum Series Lockhart Grill on SMOKE mode and let it run with lid open for 10 minutes then preheat to 325°F. If using a gas or charcoal grill, set it up for medium-low heat.
2. Melt the butter 1 tablespoon of butter and olive oil in a large skillet over medium heat. Add the onions and celery and cook, stirring frequently, until soft, 3 minutes.
3. Add the garlic and mushrooms and continue to cook for 5 minutes, until the mushrooms are slightly browned.
4. Deglaze with marsala wine, using a wooden spoon to scrape up any browned bits from the bottom of the pan.
5. Add the dried cranberries, black pepper, sage, and salt and simmer for 2 minutes, then remove from the heat.
6. Fold the stuffing into the vegetable mixture, then slowly pour over turkey stock, until stuffing is moistened.
7. Place the Honeysuckle White® Turkey Breast on a large cutting board, skin-side down, then butterfly it. Season with salt and pepper, then spoon over ⅓ of the stuffing, leaving an inch border.
8. Roll the turkey breast, starting at the side with less skin. Use butcher's twine to truss the turkey breast and secure the stuffing. Place in a cast iron skillet, top remaining butter, season with salt and pepper. Place a sprig of rosemary on top, add remaining

¼ cup of stock around the turkey, along with 1 bay leaf. Transfer to the grill.

9. Cook the turkey for 1 to 1 ½ hours, until an internal temperature of 165°F is reached.

10. Remove stuffed turkey breast from the grill, rest for 15 minutes, then slice and serve warm, with remaining stuffing.

moked Turketta (bacon Wrapped Turkey Breast)

ervings: 6

ooking Time: 180 Minutes

Ingredients:

- 1 Shady Brook Farms Turketta

Directions:

1. Fire up your Pit Boss pellet grill on SMOKE mode and let it run with lid open for 10 minutes then preheat to 250°F. If using a gas or charcoal grill, set it up for low, indirect heat.

2. Place the Turketta directly on the grill grate and smoke for 2½ to 3 hours, or until an internal temperature of 165°F is reached.

Bbq Smoked Turkey Jerky

ervings: 4 - 6

ooking Time: 120 Minutes

Ingredients:

- 2 Tablespoons Apple Cider Vinegar
- 2 Tablespoons (Any Kind) Barbecue Sauce
- 1 Tablespoon Quick Curing Salt
- ½ Cup Soy Sauce
- 4 Tablespoons Sweet Sweet Rib Rub
- 2 Pounds Boneless Skinless Turkey Breast
- ¼ Cup Water

Directions:

1. In a large bowl, combine the soy sauce, water, barbecue sauce, apple cider vinegar, quick curing salt, and 2 tablespoons of the

Sweet Rib Rub. Whisk together until well combined and pour into a large, resealable plastic bag.

2. Using a sharp knife, slice the turkey into ¼ inch slices with the grain (this is easier if the meat is partially frozen). Trim off any fat, skin or connective tissue and discard.

3. Place the turkey slices into the plastic bag, seal, and massage the marinade into the turkey. Refrigerate for 24 hours.

4. Once the jerky is ready to go, remove the turkey from the refrigerator, drain the marinade and discard. Pat the turkey dry with paper towels and sprinkle all sides generously with the remaining Sweet Rib Rub.

5. Fire up your Pit Boss Smoker and set the temperature to 180°F. If you're using a sawdust or charcoal smoker, set it up for medium low heat.

6. Place the turkey slices directly onto the smoker grates and smoke for 2-4 hours, or until the jerky is chewy but still bends slightly.

7. Transfer the jerky to a resealable plastic bag while the jerky is still warm and allow it to sit at room temperature for 1 hour. Squeeze any air from the bag and place in the refrigerator. It will keep for several weeks.

Pepper And Onion Turkey Burger Sliders

Servings: 5
Cooking Time: 30 Minutes
Ingredients:

- 1 Sweet Onion, Chopped
- 1 Pepper, Anaheim
- Pit Boss Bacon Cheddar Burger Seasoning
- Spinach
- 16 Oz Turkey, Ground

Directions:

1. Turn your grill onto smoke until the flame catches, then turn it to 400°F.
2. Put the ground turkey into a bowl and generously add the Pit Boss Bacon Cheddar Burger seasoning to the mixture.
3. Dice the Anaheim pepper and add it to the bowl as well.
4. Dice about 1/3 of the sweet onion and add it to the bowl.
5. Mix with your hands until the meat looks evenly coated in seasoning and the veggies are evenly mixed.
6. Separate the meat out into 3oz balls, disperse or toss the remnants.
7. Use the Pit Boss 3-in-1 Burger press to create the perfect patty! Place the patties on the grill and cook for 15-20 minutes depending on their thickness. Flip every 5ish minutes.
8. Add the buns to the grill if you'd like them toasted!
9. Remove the turkey sliders (and the buns) from the grill, add spinach, and whatever you think will taste good!
10. Caution: they're delicious :)

Smoked Turkey Legs

Servings: 4
Cooking Time: 150 Minutes
Ingredients:

- 1 Cup Chicken Stock
- 2 Tbsp Pit Boss Blackened Sriracha Rub
- 4 Turkey Legs (Drumsticks)

Directions:

1. Fire up your Pit Boss pellet grill on SMOKE mode. With the lid open, let it run for 10 minutes.
2. Preheat grill to 225°F. If using a gas or charcoal grill, set it up for low, indirect heat.
3. Combine turkey stock with 2 teaspoons of Pit Boss Blackened Sriracha Rub.
4. Place turkey legs on a sheet tray, then inject each with seasoned stock. Season the outside of the legs with remaining Blackened Sriracha.
5. Place turkey legs directly on the grate of the smoking cabinet, and cook for 1 ½ hours.
6. Increase temperature to 325°F, then transfer turkey legs to the bottom grill and cook for another 45 to 60 minutes, until the internal temperature reaches 170°F.
7. Remove turkey from the grill, allow to rest for 10 minutes, then serve warm.

Hot And Fast Bbq Turkey

Servings: 8
Cooking Time: 120 Minutes
Ingredients:

- 1 Bay Leaf
- 1/2 Tsp Black Peppercorns, Ground
- Pinch Chili Flakes
- 4 Garlic Cloves, Peeled And Smashed
- 1/4 Cup Honey
- 3/4 Cup Honey Chipotle Bbq Sauce
- 1 Honeysuckle White® Turkey, Thawed
- 1 Tsp Kosher Salt
- 1/4 Cup Olive Oil
- 3 Thyme Sprigs
- 1 Cup Turkey Stock
- 3 Cups Water
- 2 Tbsp Worcestershire Sauce

Directions:

1. Rinse Honeysuckle White® turkey thoroughly under cold water, then blot dry with paper towels. Place on a greased rack of a roasting pan. Set aside.
2. Prepare the injection solution: in a saucepot, whisk together the turkey stock, honey, olive oil, smashed garlic, Worcestershire sauce, salt, pepper, and chili flakes. Add in the thyme sprigs and bay leaf. Bring mixture to a boil, then simmer for 5 minutes. Remove from heat, cool for 30 minutes, then strain.
3. Using an injection needle, inject the solution throughout the turkey. Rub 1 tablespoon of solution over the top of the turkey. Add water to the bottom of the roasting pan. Set aside.
4. Fire up your Pit Boss pellet grill on SMOKE mode and let it run with lid open for 10 minutes then preheat to 450° F. If using a gas or charcoal grill, set it up for high heat.
5. Transfer the turkey to the grill and roast for 100 to 120 minutes, until an internal temperature of 165° F is reached, rotating every 30 minutes. Tent with foil after 30 minutes, then brush all over with BBQ sauce during the final 10 minutes of roasting time.
6. Remove from the grill, and allow the turkey to rest for 30 minutes, then carve and serve warm.

Bourbon Glazed Smoked Turkey Breast

Servings: 6
Cooking Time: 240 Minutes
Ingredients:
- 1/2 Tbsp Black Pepper
- 1/2 Cup Bourbon
- 1/2 Tbsp Garlic Powder
- 1 1/2 Tbsp Kosher Salt
- 1/4 Cup Maple Syrup
- 2 Tbsp Olive Oil
- 1/2 Tbsp Onion Powder
- 1/4 Cup Orange Juice
- 9 Lbs Shady Brook Farms® Turkey Breast, Whole, Bone-In
- 1 Sweet Potato, Halved
- 2 Tbsp Tamari
- 1/2 Tbsp Thyme, Dried
- 1 Yellow Onion, Halved

Directions:

1. Rinse turkey thoroughly under cold water, then blot dry with paper towels.
2. Rub turkey with olive oil, then season inside and outside of the cavity with a blend of kosher salt, black pepper, garlic powder, onion powder, and dried thyme. Place in a cast-iron skillet, and prop up on either side with onion and potato. Set aside.
3. Fire up your Pit Boss pellet grill on SMOKE mode and let it run with lid open for 10 minutes then preheat to 250° F. If using a gas or charcoal grill, set it up for low, indirect heat.
4. Transfer turkey to the grill and smoke for 3 to 3 ½ hours, or until an internal temperature of 165 F is reached, rotating after 1 ½ hours.
5. Meanwhile, prepare the glaze: melt the butter in a small saucepan, over medium heat.
6. Whisk in the bourbon, maple syrup, orange juice, and soy sauce. Bring to a boil, then reduce to a simmer.
7. Simmer for 10 minutes, until sauce begins to reduce and slightly thicken. Set aside.
8. Baste turkey with the glaze every 20 to 30 minutes, after rotating the turkey.
9. Remove the turkey from the grill and allow it to rest for 20 minutes before slicing, and serving warm.

Bbq Dry Rubbed Turkey Drumsticks

Servings: 6
Cooking Time: 120 Minutes
Ingredients:

- 1/2 Tbsp Black Pepper
- 1 Tbsp Brown Sugar
- 1/2 Tsp Cayenne Pepper
- 1/2 Tbsp Coriander, Ground
- 1/2 Tbsp Granulated Garlic
- 1 Package, Approx 4 Lbs Honeysuckle White® Turkey Drumsticks
- 1 Tbsp Kosher Salt
- 2 Tbsp Olive Oil

Directions:

1. Fire up your Pit Boss pellet grill on SMOKE mode and let it run with lid open for 10 minutes then preheat to 225°F. If using a gas or charcoal grill, set it up for low, indirect heat.
2. Place Honeysuckle White® Turkey Legs on a sheet tray, coat with olive oil, then season with a blend of salt pepper, cayenne, brown sugar, granulated garlic, and ground coriander.
3. Place turkey legs in the smoking cabinet and smoke for 1 ½ hours, checking the internal temperature after 1 hour.
4. Increase the temperature to 325°F, transfer the turkey legs to the bottom grill grate and cook for another 25 to 30 minutes, until the internal temperature reaches 170°F.
5. Remove turkey drumsticks from the grill, allow to rest for 10 minutes, then serve warm.

Sweet Heat Cajun Spatchcock Turkey

Servings: 7
Cooking Time: 180 Minutes
Ingredients:

- 16 Oz Cajun Butter
- Pit Boss Sweet Heat Rub
- 1 Brined Turkey

Directions:

1. Preheat Pit Boss Grill to 300°F
2. Inject the Turkey with Cajun butter and season liberally with Pit Boss Sweet Heat Rub.
3. Place on the grill and cook until thighs and breasts reach 165°.
4. Let rest for 30 minutes and serve.

Maple Smoked Thanksgiving Turkey

Servings: 8
Cooking Time: 375 Minutes
Ingredients:

- 1 Cup Butter, Room Temp
- 1/2 Cup Maple Syrup
- 2 Tablespoons Pit Boss Champion Chicken Seasoning
- 1, (Pre-Brined) Turkey, Whole

Directions:

1. Start your Grill on "smoke" with the lid open until a fire is established in the burn pot (3-7 minutes).
2. Preheat to 250°F degrees.
3. Combine the melted butter and maple syrup in a bowl. With the Marinade Injector, fill with the butter and syrup mixture and pierce the meat with the needle while pushing on the plunger, injecting the flavor. You want to inject the marinade into the thickest part of the breast, thigh, and wings.
4. Next, combine the room temperature butter and Champion Chicken seasoning and spread all over the turkey, making sure that you get it under the skin as well.
5. Place the turkey in an aluminum pan to catch all the drippings (this makes incredible gravy) and place on the grill.

6. When the breast and thigh meat of the turkey reaches 165°F to 170°F, remove from grill and let rest 15 minutes before carving. Happy Thanksgiving!

Bacon Lattice Turkey

Servings: 7

Cooking Time: 180 Minutes

Ingredients:

- 2 Apples
- Bacon
- 2 Celery, Stick
- (Parsley, Rosemary, Thyme) Herb Mix
- 1 Onion, Sliced
- Pepper
- Pit Boss Grills Champion Chicken Seasoning
- 1 Brined Turkey

Directions:

1. Preheat grill to 300°F.
2. Be sure all the innards and giblets of the turkey have been removed.
3. Wash the external and internal parts of the turkey and pat the surface dry with a paper towel.
4. Slice fruit and veggies into large chunks and stuff inside turkey.
5. Liberally season the whole Turkey with Champion Chicken Seasoning.
6. Prep bacon into lattice design on a flexible cutting board. Flip onto top of turkey, covering the breasts.
7. Season with more Champion Chicken and black pepper
8. Season with more Champion Chicken and black pepper
9. Let the turkey rest for 30 minutes.

Teriyaki Glazed Whole Turkey

Servings: 8-10

Cooking Time: 180 Minutes

Ingredients:

- 1/2 Cup Apple Cider
- 1/4 Cup Melted Butter, Unsalted
- 1 Teaspoon Cornstarch
- 2 Finely Chopped Garlic, Cloves
- 1/2 Teaspoon Ginger, Ground
- 2 Tablespoon Honey
- 2 Tablespoon Pit Boss Champion Chicken Seasoning
- 1 Shady Brook Farms® Whole Turkey, Thawed
- 2 Tablespoon Soy Sauce
- 1 Tablespoon Water, Cold

Directions:

1. Turn your Pit Boss grill to smoke mode, let the fire catch and then set to 300°F.
2. In a saucepan, whisk together melted butter, garlic, soy sauce, apple cider, ground ginger, and honey. Bring to a boil then reduce to a simmer.
3. Place the turkey in an aluminum roasting pan.
4. With a marinade injector, fill with the mixture and pierce the meat with the needle while pushing on the plunger, injecting the flavor. You want to inject into the thickest part of the breast, thigh, and wings.
5. Next, rub entire turkey with your favorite poultry seasoning or the Pit Boss Champion Chicken seasoning. For added flavor, throw some extra garlic gloves into the cavity and apple cider in the aluminum pan.
6. Place the turkey in the grill and cook until the internal temperature reaches 165-170°F.
7. In a separate bowl, mix cornstarch and cold water together and add to the leftover original mixture to create a glaze. Glaze the turkey with the remaining mixture with approximately 15-20 minutes left. Skin will darken because of the sugar in the glaze.

8. Let the turkey rest 20-25 minutes before carving and enjoy!

Smoked Turkey Tamale Pie

Servings: 6
Cooking Time: 240 Minutes
Ingredients:

- 1 Avocado, Diced (For Topping)
- 15 Oz Black Beans, Drained (For Filling)
- To Taste, Blackened Sriracha Rub Seasoning
- 2 Tsp Blackened Sriracha Rub Seasoning (For Filling)
- To Taste, Blackened Sriracha Rub Seasoning (For Polenta)
- 2 Tbsp Butter (For Polenta)
- 2 Tbsp Cilantro, Chopped (For Topping)
- 1 Cup Corn Kernels (For Filling)
- 2 Cups Enchilada Sauce (For Filling)
- 1/2 Jalapeño, Minced (For Topping)
- 2 Cups Milk Or Water (For Polenta)
- 1 Cup Polenta, Or Fine Cornmeal (For Polenta)
- 2 Scallions, Sliced (For Topping)
- 2 Cups Smoked Turkey Breast, Shredded (For Filling)
- 2 1/2 Lbs Split Turkey Breast , Bone-In
- 2 Cups Turkey Stock (For Polenta)
- 4 Oz White Cheddar, Shredded (For Polenta)
- 4 Oz White Cheddar, Shredded (For Topping)

Directions:
1. Fire up your Pit Boss Platinum Series KC Combo on SMOKE mode and let it run with lid open for 10 minutes then preheat to 225° F. If using a gas or charcoal grill, set it up for low, indirect heat.
2. Season the turkey breast with Blackened Sriracha, then transfer to the grill, on a rack, over indirect heat.
3. Smoke the turkey breast for 2 ½ to 3 hours, until an internal temperature of 16 F. Remove the turkey from the grill, allow to rest for 20 minutes, then shred with 2 forks.
4. While the turkey is resting, prepare the polenta:
5. Place a deep, cast iron skillet on the grill, then increase the temperature to 375° F. Add chicken broth and milk to a skillet and bring to a boil.
6. Whisk in the polenta, then reduce the hea to a simmer, stirring often for 5 minutes. Season with Blackened Sriracha, then stir in cheese and butter. Remove the skillet from the grill and smooth out the polenta in an even layer.
7. In a large glass measuring cup or mixing bowl, combine the turkey, enchilada sauc black beans, corn and Blackened Sriracha
8. Spoon the turkey mixture over the polent then top with 4 ounces of shredded chees Place on the grill, over indirect heat and bake for 20 to 25 minutes, until the filling is bubbling along the edge and the cheese is melted.
9. Remove the skillet from the grill and allow it to rest for 10 minutes. Serve warm, garnished with avocado, scallions, jalapeño, and fresh cilantro.

Brie Stuffed Turkey Burgers

Servings: 9

Cooking Time: 25 Minutes

Ingredients:

- Blueberry Jalapeno Spread
- 7Oz Bar Brie Cheese
- Burger Buns
- Pit Boss Sweet Onion Burger Seasoning
- 1 Or 2 Red Bell Peppers
- Spinach
- 3 Lbs Turkey, Ground

Directions:

1. Slice the brie into pieces, roughly about 1/2in Wx1in H. (It's ok if they aren't all even, you can puzzle piece them together in the burger as needed, so don't go crazy with measuring this!)

2. Put the 3lbs of ground turkey into a mixing bowl, generously cover with Sweet Onion Burger Seasoning (seasoning amount to preference). Mix the seasoning into the turkey, add additional seasoning if desired.

3. Once the seasoning is mixed into the ground turkey, portion the meat out into 1/3lb balls. Using the Burger Press, add half of the burger patty into the bottom of the press, then add about 3 pieces of cheese to the center of the meat. Place the remaining half of the burger patty on top of the cheese. Press the burger a couple times using the Burger Press and voil. Flip the press to remove your burger! (repeat)

4. Note: you don't want to see a bunch of the cheese sticking out of the burger patty, make sure it is mostly covered by the meat, in the center, so it doesn't get cooked off on the grill.

5. Remove the burgers from the grill and make your creation! The sweet and spicy jam adds a lot of flavor to the burger, but whatever kind of preserve you want to add is your call, Boss.

VEGGIES RECIPES

Hasselback Potato Bites

Servings: 4
Cooking Time: 40 Minutes

Ingredients:

- Cheese, Sliced
- Olive Oil
- 1 Lb Potato, Baby
- Salt, Kosher

Directions:

1. Start your Grill on "smoke" with the lid open until a fire is established in the burn pot (3-7 minutes).
2. Preheat to 400F.
3. Place all ingredients in a bowl, combine them and stir well.
4. Shape the mixture into 30 meatballs (1 ½ inches in width).
5. Spray a broiler pan with cooking spray, place on the grill, and bake for 15 minutes until fully cooked and browned.
6. Remove from grill, cool for 5 minutes, and serve.

Parmesan Crusted Smashed Potatoes

Servings: 4
Cooking Time: 10 Minutes

Ingredients:

- 3 Tbsp Butter, Melted
- To Taste Cracked Black Pepper
- 1/4 Tsp Garlic, Granulated
- 1/3 Cup Parmesan Cheese
- 1 Tbsp Parsley, Leaves
- 2 Lbs, Yukon Gold Potatoes
- To Taste Salt
- 2 Tbsp Vegetable Oil

Directions:

1. Fire up your Pit Boss Platinum Series KC Combo and preheat the griddle to medium-low flame. If using a gas or charcoal grill, preheat a large cast iron skillet over medium-low heat.
2. Evenly distribute the cooled potatoes on a metal sheet tray, drizzle with olive oil, and use a potato masher or small metal bowl to gently smash each potato to a height of about ¼ to ½ inch (thinner potatoes will be crispier).
3. Mix together the butter and garlic. Brush the mixture over each potato, then season with salt and pepper.
4. Pour vegetable oil on griddle, then add flattened potatoes. Cook for 3 minutes, then flip and sprinkle with half of Parmesan. Cook for 3 minutes, then flip, sprinkle with remaining Parmesan, and cook 1 minute.
5. Transfer to a pan, sprinkle with parsley and serve hot.

Grilled Potato Salad With Smoked Hard Boiled Eggs

Servings: 6
Cooking Time: 60 Minutes

Ingredients:

- 1/2 Cup Bacon Bits
- 8 Peeled Egg, Boiled
- 1 Cup Mayonnaise
- 1 Tbsp Olive Oil
- 1/4 Cup Parsley, Chopped
- Tt Pit Boss Hickory Bacon Rub
- 3 Scallions, Chopped
- 1 Cup Sour Cream
- 2 Tbsp Spicy Brown Mustard
- 2 Lbs Yukon Gold Potatoes

Directions:

1. Fire up your Pit Boss Platinum Series Lockhart and preheat to 275°F. If using a gas or charcoal grill, set it up for low, indirect heat.
2. Drizzle olive oil over potatoes. Season both potatoes and eggs with Hickory Bacon.

3. Place potatoes over indirect heat on the grill grate. Place eggs in the smoking cabinet, directly on grates. Remove after 1 hour.
4. Allow potatoes to cool for 10 minutes, then cut in half and return to grill and place flesh side down over direct flame for 1 minute. Remove from grill and cool.
5. Meanwhile, prepare dressing in a mixing bowl by whisking together mayonnaise, sour cream, mustard, bacon bits, parsley, and scallions.
6. Quarter potatoes and cut eggs in half then quarter. Gently mix potatoes and eggs into dressing. Refrigerate for 1 hour, then serve.

Grilled Sweet Potato Casserole

Servings: 4
Cooking Time: 90 Minutes
Ingredients:

- 1/4 Cup Brown Sugar
- Butter, Softened
- 4 Oz Chopped Pecans
- ½ Tsp Cinnamon
- 6 Oz. Mini Marshmallows
- 2 Tsp Pit Boss Tennessee Apple Butter Rub
- 4 Sweet Potatoes

Directions:

1. Fire up your Pit Boss and preheat to 400° F. If using a gas or charcoal grill, set it for medium-high heat.
2. Wash and scrub potatoes then pat dry with paper towel.
3. Coat outside of potatoes generously in softened butter then set butter aside. Place the sweet potatoes directly on the grill grate and smoke until soft, 1 to 1 ½ hours depending on the size of your sweet potatoes.
4. Once sweet potatoes are soft remove from the grill. Coat with more butter and cover with brown sugar and Tennessee Apple Butter. Slice the center of the sweet potato and press on the sides to create an opening. Stuff each sweet potato with a layer of butter, brown sugar, cinnamon, chopped pecans, and marshmallows.
5. Return to the grill and cook, covered, for five minutes, or until marshmallows are lightly browned. Remove from grill and serve warm.

Braised Collard Greens

Servings: 4
Cooking Time: 45 Minutes
Ingredients:

- 2 Quarts Broth, Chicken
- 3 Lbs, Woody Stems Removed And Cut Into Thick Ribbons Collard Greens
- 4 Peeled Garlic, Cloves
- 3 Smoked Ham Hock
- For Serving Hot Pepper Vinegar
- 2 Whole Yellow Onion, Sliced
- To Taste Salt And Pepper
- 2 Tbsp Sweet Heat Rub

Directions:

1. In a large stock pot, combine the chicken broth, Sweet Heat Rub, sliced onions, garlic and ham hocks. Cover and simmer for 2-3 hours, or until the ham hocks are tender. Allow to cool.
2. Remove the meat from the ham hocks and chop. Add the collard greens to the broth, fully submerged, and simmer for 30-45 minutes, or until the greens are tender.
3. Season to taste, add vinegar if desired, and enjoy!

Brussels Sprout Slaw With Apple Butter Dressing

Servings: 6-8

Cooking Time: 10 Minutes

Ingredients:

- 1/4 Cup (For Apple Butter Dressing) Apple Butter
- 2 Tablespoon (For Apple Butter Dressing) Apple Cider Vinegar
- 8 (For The Slaw) Bacon, Strip
- 2 Lbs (For The Slaw) Brussels Sprouts, Rinsed And Trimmed
- 1/2 Teaspoon (For Apple Butter Dressing) Chipotle Pepper, Ground
- 1 Teaspoon (For Apple Butter Dressing) Cinnamon, Ground
- 1/2 Teaspoon (For Apple Butter Dressing) Coriander, Ground
- 1 Cup (For Apple Butter Dressing) Olive Oil
- 1 (For Apple Butter Dressing) Orange, Zest
- 1/2 Cup (For The Slaw) Parmesan Cheese, Shredded
- 1/2 Cup (For The Slaw) Pecans, Toasted
- 1 Teaspoon (For Apple Butter Dressing) Pit Boss Applewood Smoked Bacon Seasoning
- 1/4 Cup (For The Slaw) Pomegranate Arils
- 1 (For The Slaw) Yellow Onion
- Yellow Onion, Sliced

Directions:

1. For the slaw: in a food processor, fit the bowl with a medium grating blade. Shred the brussels sprouts and set aside.
2. Place the bacon and yellow on a grill basket and season both sides with Pit Boss Applewood Smoked Bacon Seasoning. Turn your Pit Boss Grill to 350F and grill for 5-10 minutes, or until bacon is crispy and the yellow onion is soft. Remove from grill and chop into ¼ inch pieces. Set aside.
3. For the dressing: in a large bowl, whisk together the oil, apple butter, coriander, chipotle pepper, cinnamon, vinegar, orange zest and Applewood Smoked Bacon seasoning. Whisk to combine.
4. To assemble the salad: in a large salad bowl, stir together the shredded brussels sprouts, chopped pecans, chopped bacon, parmesan cheese, pomegranate arils and dressing. Serve and enjoy!

Roasted Pineapple Salsa

Servings: 4

Cooking Time: 30 Minutes

Ingredients:

- Cilantro
- 1 Large Onion, Diced
- 1 Pineapple, Chopped
- 1 Tbsp Pit Boss Mandarin Habanero Spice
- 1 Red Bell Peppers
- 5 Tomato, Roma
- 1 Bag Tortilla Chip

Directions:

1. Set your Grill to 250°F and roast the vegetables whole for 30 minutes. Use Hickory Pellets for your wood pellet grill, to give it a 100% hardwood smoke.
2. While the vegetables are roasting on your Grill, split a whole Pineapple and make a bowl out of one side. Remove the core and place the leftover diced pineapple in a bowl along with some freshly diced cilantro.
3. Once the vegetables are done roasting, peel the tomatoes. Dice the roasted onion, red peppers, and tomatoes. Place in bowl.
4. Add a tablespoon of Mandarin Habanero and process with a hand blender to a chunky consistency.
5. Make some Guacamole with the extra roasted tomatoes and onions.
6. Serve with Nachos!

Corn On The Cob

Servings: 6
Cooking Time: 20 Minutes
Ingredients:

- 1/2 Cup Butter, Melted
- 6 Corn, Cob
- Salt

Directions:

1. Preheat your Grill to 400 degrees F.
2. Husk the corn and be sure to remove all the silk. Brush with melted butter and sprinkle with salt.
3. Place the corn on the grates of your grill, and rotate every 5 minutes until your desired level of golden brown is achieved. Brush with butter halfway through (or as much as you feel - the more the better).
4. Serve warm. Enjoy!

Scalloped Potatoes

Servings: 10
Cooking Time: 90 Minutes
Ingredients:

- 1 L Heavy Cream
- 2 Cups Mozzarella Cheese, Shredded
- 1 Onion, Sliced
- 8 Red Potatoes, Sliced

Directions:

1. Preheat your Grill to 350F.
2. In a large cast iron pan, layer potatoes and onion. Pour in heavy cream until all potatoes are covered except the top layer. Sprinkle on cheese.
3. Bake in your uncovered for about 1 ½ hour, with the lid closed. The cheese should be golden brown and potatoes soft. Serve hot. Enjoy!

Lemon Garlic Green Beans

Servings: 6
Cooking Time: 20 Minutes
Ingredients:

- 3 - 5 Tbs Butter
- 3 Garlic, Cloves
- 1 Lb Green Bean, Whole
- Pepper
- Pit Boss Lemon Pepper Garlic Seasoning
- Salt

Directions:

1. Turn your grill to smoke, once the fire pot catches - preheat your grill to 350° F.
2. Melt the butter in a ramekin.
3. While your grill is heating, line the grilling basket with tinfoil. Add the green beans and melted butter.
4. Add salt, pepper, and Pit Boss Grills Lemon Pepper Garlic Seasoning to taste
5. Add 2-3 cloves of minced garlic.
6. Toss all ingredients until evenly mixed.
7. Place basket on the grill and cook for 15-20 minutes. Toss the basket half way through the cook time.
8. Once your lemon garlic green beans are finished, remove them and add them to a serving dish – contents are hot! Caution as the butter may boil, splatter a bit.

Grilled Garlic Potatoes

Servings: 6
Cooking Time: 30 Minutes
Ingredients:

- 3 Tbsp Butter
- 3 Sliced Garlic, Cloves
- 1 Large Onion, Sliced
- 1 Tsp Chopped Parsley, Leaves
- Red Potato, Baby
- 1 Cup Shredded Cheddar Cheese

Directions:

1. Preheat the grill then increase the temperature to 400°F.
2. Cut and arrange potato slices, separated by onion and butter slices, on a large piece of commercial grade aluminum foil. If commercial grade aluminum foil is

unavailable, layer aluminum foil until it is strong, or use a baking sheet.

3. Top potatoes with garlic, and season with parsley, salt, and pepper. Place potatoes on the aluminum foil.

4. Place on the preheated grill and cook for 30-40 minutes or until potatoes are tender. Serve hot.

5. an option, you can sprinkle potatoes with shredded cheddar cheese, reseal foil packets, and continue cooking 5 minutes, or until cheese is melted.

Mexican Street Corn Salad

Servings: 4
Cooking Time: 10 Minutes
Ingredients:
- 1 Tablespoon Of Chopped Cilantro
- 4 Corn, Cob
- 1/2 Cup Crumbled Feta Cheese
- 1 Lime, Juiced
- 2 Tablespoon Mayo
- 1 Teaspoon Paprika, Smoked
- 1 Tablespoon Pit Boss Champion Chicken Seasoning
- 1/4 Cup Sour Cream

Directions:
1. Preheat your Pit Boss Grill to 350F. Grill the corn cobs until slightly charred on all sides, about 10 minutes. Remove from the grill and allow to cool.

2. Remove the kernels of corn from the cob and set aside. In a separate bowl, mix together the sour cream, mayonnaise, lime juice, Champion Chicken seasoning, smoked paprika, and cilantro until smooth. Mix with the corn and feta cheese, then serve immediately.

Gluten Free Mashed Potato Cakes

Servings: 6
Cooking Time: 10 Minutes
Ingredients:
- 1/2 Cup Bacon Bits
- 2 Tbsp Butter
- 1 Cup Cheddar Jack Cheese, Shredded
- 1 Egg, Whisked
- 1/3 Cup Flour, Gluten Free
- 3 Cups Mashed Potatoes, Prepared
- 1 Tsp Pit Boss Hickory Bacon Rub
- 4 Scallions, Minced
- 2 Tsp Spicy Mustard

Directions:
1. In a mixing bowl, combine mashed potatoes, bacon bits, scallions, mustard, cheddar jack cheese, and beaten egg. In a separate bowl, whisk together flour, and teaspoon of Pit Boss Hickory Bacon Rub. Incorporate dry into wet ingredients. Cover and refrigerate for 30 minutes.

2. Remove mixture from the refrigerator, then divide into 12 balls (about 2 ½ inches in diameter), and set on a greased sheet tray. Use the bottom of a bowl to press down each potato ball to form a ½ inch thick patty. Season with additional sprinkling of Hickory Bacon and set aside. Fire up your Pit Boss Platinum Series KC Combo or Pit Boss Griddle and preheat the griddle to medium-low flame. If using a gas or charcoal grill, preheat a cast iron skillet over medium-low heat.

3. Add butter and oil to griddle to melt, then place mashed potato cakes on the griddle. Cook for 2 to 3 minutes per side, until golden brown.

4. Remove from the griddle. Serve warm with sour cream, reserved bacon bits and scallions.

Hickory Smoked Chive And Cheese Twice Baked Sweet Potatoes

Servings: 6

Cooking Time: 60 Minutes

Ingredients:

- 3 Pieces Brown Sugar Bacon
- Chives, Chopped
- 1 Cup Colby Jack Cheese, Shredded
- 2 Tbs Olive Oil
- Pit Boss Hickory Smoked Finishing Salt
- 3 Potato, Sweet
- 2 Tbs Sour Cream

Directions:

1. Turn your grill to smoke, once the fire pot catches - preheat your grill to 400° F.
2. Washing sweet potatoes and rub olive oil on the skins. Poke holes in the potatoes with a fork.
3. Once grill is heated add bacon rack with brown Sugar bacon – cook 10-15 minutes
4. Place sweet potatoes on indirect flame/heat and cook for about 50 minutes.
5. Remove sweet potatoes and let cool.
6. Reduce the heat to 350° F (for when you put the potatoes back on the grill).
7. While cooling add the sour cream, cheese, 2 tbs(ish) of diced chives, and crumbled bacon into a mixing bowl.
8. Once the potatoes have cooled enough to touch, cut them in half lengthwise.
9. Scoop out the insides with a spoon and add them to the mixing bowl, leaving enough potato to create a boat-like shell.
10. Mix the ingredients together, sprinkle with Pit Boss Grill Hickory Smoked Salt, and add them back into the potato skins.
11. Top with additional shredded cheese or chives if desired.
12. Place the potatoes on a backing sheet, covered with parchment paper (to help prevent burning).
13. Bake for 15-20 minutes, or until the cheese is melted and the tops slightly brown.
14. Remove from the grill and let cool briefly. Top with additional sour cream, some butter, or bacon if desired! Eat up!!

Smoked Scalloped Potatoes

Servings: 4-6
Cooking Time: 60 Minutes
Ingredients:

- 1 Stick Of Butter
- Cast Iron Skillet Or Pan
- 1/2 Chedder Jack Or Colby Jack Cheese, Shredded
- Medium Yellow Onion
- Pit Boss Bacon Cheddar Seasoning
- 6-8 Potatoes
- Salt And Pepper
- Smoked Guoda Cheese, Sliced

Directions:

1. Preheat Grill to 350°F.
2. Peel 6-8 potatoes and slice into 1/4 round slices, cover with water in pot and bring to boil, allow to boil for 2-3 minutes.
3. In the cast iron skillet, start to layer the potatoes and cheese. Starting by using a slotted spoon to remove potatoes from water. You will want some of the water from the boiling process to make it int the skillet, but not an excessive amount. Using a slotted spoon but not shaking the potatoes dry works perfectly.
4. Once you have a base layer of potatoes, add a layer of sliced onion (approx. ½ of a medium yellow onion), salt, pepper, Pit Boss Bacon Cheddar Burger Seasoning, a drizzle of sweet condensed milk, half a stick of butter cut into pats, and a layer of sliced smoked gouda cheese.
5. Repeat on the 2nd layer. Top with grated cheddar jack or Colby jack cheese.
6. Cook at 325°F-350°F for approx. 1 hour or until the potatoes are tender.
7. For crustier cheese on top, turn the grill up to 425°F for the last 10 to 15 minutes or until the cheese is golden brown.

Simply Bossin' Tortilla Chips

Servings: 4
Cooking Time: 15 Minutes
Ingredients:

- Olive Oil
- Pit Boss Cilantro Lime Seasoning
- 8 Flour Tortilla

Directions:

1. Preheat your Grill to 350F.
2. Drizzle olive oil over each flour tortilla. Sprinkle with Cilantro Lime Seasoning and cut into triangles Place on a prepared baking sheet and grill for 15 minutes. Serve with salsa or your favorite hot dip!

Chili Verde Sauce

Servings: 4

Cooking Time: 10 Minutes

Ingredients:

- 1 Cup Cilantro
- 3 Cloves Garlic, Peeled
- 1 Medium Onion, Peeled And Quartered
- ¼ Cup Olive Oil
- 3-4 Serrano Chili Pepper, Halved And Seeded
- 1 Tbsp Sweet Heat Rub
- 1 Lb. Tomatillos, Husks Removed

Directions:

1. Fire up your pellet grill and set the temperature to 350°F. If you're using a gas or charcoal grill, set it up for medium high heat. In a bowl, toss the tomatillos, onion, garlic, and peppers with the oil and toss to coat evenly.
2. Grill vegetables until slight charred and bubbling on all sides, about 10 – 20 minutes. Remove from grill and allow to cool slightly.
3. Transfer grilled vegetables to a blender and add the cilantro, lime juice, olive oil, and Sweet Heat Rub. Pulse the ingredients until they have a consistent texture to them.

Sweet Potato Medley

Servings: 6-8

Cooking Time: 45 Minutes

Ingredients:

- 8-10 Brussels Sprouts
- 2-3 Tablespoons Olive Oil
- 1/2 Sweet White Softball Sized White Onion
- 1 Red Bell Pepper
- Pit Boss Lemon Pepper Garlic Seasoning
- 2 Sweet Potatoes, Scrubbed

Directions:

1. Slice the sweet potatoes, and then cut them into quarters. Slice the onion, Anaheim pepper and bell pepper. Be sure to make these slices big enough that they won't fall though the holes in your Pit Boss Grilling Basket. Cut the brussels sprouts vertically, stems at the bottom, in 1/2 or 1/3's depending on their size.
2. Add the sweet potatoes to your grilling basket. Drizzle olive oil, enough to cover the potatoes, but not enough to drown them. Sprinkle with Pit Boss Lemon Pepper Garlic seasoning (to taste), and toss again.

3. Toss or mix the additional vegetables in a bowl, and drizzle olive oil over these as well so they are evenly covered with the olive oil. Set aside.
4. Preheat your grill to 450F.
5. Place the sweet potatoes on the grill, (indirect flame heating). Your Medley will take 45-50 minutes depending on the thickness of your potatoes.
6. Every 15 minutes, go out to your Pit Boss Grill and toss/mix the potatoes. After 30 minutes, add the rest of the vegetables to the potatoes and toss - so that the Medley cooks evenly.
7. When finished, remove the vegetables from the grill, and add them to a serving bowl. Serve hot, and chow down!

Cinnamon Twice Baked Sweet Potatoes

Servings: 6
Cooking Time: 60 Minutes
Ingredients:
- 3 Pieces Brown Sugar Bacon
- 3 Tbs Butter
- 1 Tsp Cinnamon, Ground
- (Optional) Marshmallow, Mini
- 1/2 Tsp Nutmeg, Ground
- 2 Tbs Olive Oil
- 3 Potato, Sweet

Directions:
1. Turn your grill to smoke, once the fire pot catches - preheat your grill to 400° F.
2. Washing sweet potatoes and rub olive oil on the skins. Poke holes in the potatoes with a fork.
3. Once grill is heated add bacon rack with brown Sugar bacon – cook 10-15 minutes
4. Place sweet potatoes on indirect flame/heat and cook for about 50 minutes.
5. Remove sweet potatoes and let cool.
6. Reduce the heat to 350° F (for when you put the potatoes back on the grill).
7. While cooling add the cinnamon, nutmeg, and softened butter into a mixing bowl.
8. Once the potatoes have cooled enough to touch, cut them in half lengthwise.
9. Scoop out the insides with a spoon and add them to the mixing bowl, leaving enough potato to create a boat-like shell.
10. Mix the ingredients together and add them back into the potato skins.
11. Top with bacon pieces or mini marshmallows if desired!
12. Place the potatoes on a backing sheet, covered with parchment paper (to help prevent burning).
13. Bake for 15-20 minutes, or until the tops of the marshmellows have browned.
14. Remove from the grill and let cool briefly.
15. Dig in!

Green Chile Mashed Potatoes

Servings: 4

Cooking Time: 40 Minutes

Ingredients:

- 1 Stick Butter, Unsalted
- 1 Can Green Chiles, Drained
- 1/4 - 1/2 Warm Milk, Whole
- Pit Boss Competition Smoked Rub
- 2 Tablespoon Pit Boss Competition Smoked Seasoning
- 3 Lbs Russet Potatoes, Peeled And Cut (Large Chunks)

Directions:

1. For the mashed potatoes: add the potatoes to a large pot and add enough cold water to cover the potatoes. Bring to a simmer over medium heat until the potatoes are tender enough to be pierced with a fork, about 30-35 minutes. Drain the potatoes.
2. Add the potatoes to a large mixing bowl. Add the butter, Competition Smoked Seasoning, drained green chiles and ¼ cup of warm milk. Mash until smooth and lump free. If potatoes are too thick, add more milk, a tablespoon at a time, until you reach your desired consistency.
3. Serve and enjoy!

Southern Green Beans

Servings: 6

Cooking Time: 60 Minutes

Ingredients:

- 1 Tablespoon Butter, Unsalted
- 2 Cups Chicken Broth
- 2 Pounds Green Beans, Ends Snapped Off And Longer Beans Snapped In Half
- Hickory Bacon Seasoning
- 4 Slices Bacon, Raw
- 2 Cups Water

Directions:

1. Fire up your Pit Boss grill and set the temperature to 350°F. If you're using a gas or charcoal grill, se it up for medium heat. Place a cast iron pan on the grill to preheat. Once the pan finishes preheating place the 4 slices of bacon in the pan and cook for 15 minutes until the bacon has rendered and is crispy.
2. Remove the bacon from the pan and reserve for later. Leave the pan and drippings on the grill, and add the green beans, chicken broth, water, and Hickory Bacon seasoning to taste. Close the lid on th grill and cook for an hour, or until the beans are tender.
3. Chop the bacon on a cutting board and mix into the beans with the butter. Allow the beans to cook for another minute, then remove from the heat and serve.

CPSIA information can be obtained
at www.ICGtesting.com
Printed in the USA
LVHW051435190621
690452LV00004B/36

9 781801 662857